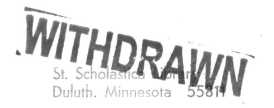

The Science and Practice of Gerontology

The Science and Practice of Gerontology

A MULTIDISCIPLINARY GUIDE

EDITED BY

Nancy J. Osgood

AND

Ann H.L. Sontz

Foreword by T. Franklin Williams

GREENWOOD PRESS

New York • Westport, Connecticut • London

Library of Congress Cataloging-in-Publication Data

The Science and practice of gerontology : a multidisciplinary guide /
   edited by Nancy J. Osgood and Ann H.L. Sontz.
       p. cm.
       Includes bibliographies and index.
       ISBN 0–313–26161–X (lib. bdg. : alk. paper)
       1. Gerontology. 2. Gerontology—United States. I. Osgood, Nancy
J. II. Sontz, Ann H.L.
   HQ1061.S326 1989
   305.2′6—dc19   88–25100

British Library Cataloguing in Publication Data is available.

Library of Congress Catalog Card Number: 88–25100
ISBN: 0–313–26161–X

First published in 1989

Greenwood Press, Inc.
88 Post Road West, Westport, Connecticut 06881

Printed in the United States of America

∞

The paper used in this book complies with the
Permanent Paper Standard issued by the National
Information Standards Organization (Z39.48–1984).

10 9 8 7 6 5 4 3 2 1

Copyright Acknowledgments

Grateful acknowledgment is made to the following publishers for permission to
quote from their works:
Brooks/Cole Publishing Company, for permission to quote from J.J. Dowd,
Stratification Among the Aged, 1980; Cornell University Press, for permission
to quote from Barbara Myerhoff, ''Rites and Signs of Ripening: The
Intertwining of Ritual, Time, and Growing Older,'' *Age and Anthropological
Theory*, edited by David I. Kertzer and Jennie Keith. Copyright © 1984 by
Cornell University Press. Used by permission of the publisher; Macmillan
Publishing Company, New York, and Routledge and Kegan Paul, Ltd.,
London, for permission to quote from A.R. Radcliffe-Brown, *Structure and
Function in Primitive Society*, 1952; and the University of California Press, for
permission to quote from Gaylene Becker, *Growing Old in Silence: Deaf
People in Old Age*, 1983.

CONTENTS

Part II. The Practicing Disciplines

ILLUSTRATIONS

FIGURES

TABLES

FOREWORD

The fact that we are all moving swiftly into the era of the aging society is by now understood widely. Scholars, teachers, health professionals, political leaders, and the lay public are all aware of the rapidly increasing numbers and percentages of older and very old persons in our country and indeed worldwide. We are well aware, too, of some of the resulting opportunities as well as the concerns for essentially all aspects of society, and we are eager to see that knowledge about all facets of the aging phenomena is extended and used.

Following limited, albeit important, early studies in the field of aging, the past ten to twenty years have seen the almost explosive growth of research and writing on gerontology (the science of aging) and its health-targeted companion field, geriatrics. This book is aimed at extending our understanding of these fields through authoritative presentations and perspectives directed at students new to aging, at students and teachers in other fields who want a broad overview, and at professionals who can find in its chapters useful insights for their practices.

The Science and Practice of Gerontology addresses a wide range of fields, from basic biological, psychological, and sociological perspectives of aging to applications in social work and medicine. Two important features characterize the contributions of the author(s) of each chapter: an historical approach leading up to the current frontiers in her/his field and an emphasis on the essential interrelations with the other fields that recognizes the unavoidable interdisciplinary nature of the study of aging and the care of older people.

With the range of descriptive knowledge now available, we should be ready to proceed with interventional efforts, to test further possible cause-and-effect relationships, and to evaluate preventive and therapeutic approaches.

I believe and hope that the audience for whom this volume is intended will find it a worthwhile introduction to the challenges of gerontology and will want to go further, in study and in research, to help us all to understand and benefit "our future selves."

T. Franklin Williams, M.D.
Director
National Institute on Aging

PREFACE

This volume was originally conceived as a reference work for the variety of professionals now engaged in research and practice with the elderly. Any reference work, however, must ultimately strive to be inclusive as well as exclusive in intent—to be a general place, as the Oxford English Dictionary would have it, "where information may be found." We hope, therefore, that this collection of articles will find a home among those who are just approaching the study of gerontology, as well as a secure place within the libraries of established scholars and practitioners. It is also our hope that the work will be adopted as a major or supplementary text in foundations and survey courses in gerontology.

A few terms warrant attention at the outset. We have used *gerontology* in our title to refer to the science of and associated practice with the elderly. Thus, the reader will find articles on the psychological, social, and cultural domains affecting older people, but also those containing general biomedical understandings and practical/clinical applications. This means that, to some extent, geriatrics has fallen within our net, even though this term is usually reserved for a specific medical subspecialty dealing with clinical practice among older adults.

Having stated this, it remains true today that gerontology still represents less a distinct academic specialization than an area focus within a variety of already established fields. By *multidisciplinary guide* in the title, then, we have necessarily implied a series of reviews of past and ongoing work in gerontology in those many theoretical and practicing disciplines where this area focus has increasingly begun to corner its share of intellectual interests and energies.

In the chapters that follow, authors broadly outline past, present, and future issues of theory, research, and practice in their particular area of interest and specialization in aging. Among the types of interesting academic issues the reader will find discussed are: crosscultural perspectives on age and aging; past and future trends in life expectancy with underlying explanations; innovations and advances in research design and methodology in the study of the aging process and the effects of age as a variable; and past and current theoretical perspectives on the psychology and sociology of aging. Some concerns relevant to practitioners and clinicians to be addressed include: successful counseling therapies with older adults; practical implications of various legislative measures such as the Older Americans Act of 1965; changes in social work and rehabilitation practice with the elderly, and newest trends and developments in each area; current and future manpower needs and research granting decisions in relation to aging research and practice; and past, present, and possible future relationships between geriatrics and gerontology, medicine and academia. Many authors underscore the historical context in which gerontology as a science and a practice discipline has developed. In combination, the chapters provide a wide-sweeping, multidisciplinary guide to a rapidly expanding field of interest.

There is little doubt that a reading of these reviews will amply indicate the rising number of significant efforts within gerontological studies now being derived from diverse disciplinary roots. Similarly present, however, is the call for those active in gerontology to identify with more than one common name, i.e., one will encounter here both a hope as well as some evidence for the emergence of actual multidisciplinary work—in the sense of a true interdisciplinary penetration of ideas and their creative usage within equally interdisciplinary social organizations and professionalized helping networks. There is, in other words, a definite desire among the contributors to evolve a theoretical and related applied arena of endeavor that is more than a refraction of single disciplinary trajectories containing a similar thematic base.

Of course, this multidisciplinary imperative speaks, in a more encompassing vein, to issues familiar to scientific history—how to reconcile tensions of an intellectual and institutional nature that arise, on the one hand, from the activities of many historically anchored disciplines and, on the other hand, from the intense need of a newly professionalizing field to evolve its own academic independence as well as a pathway toward theoretical synthesis (Kuhn, 1970). Such tensions cannot be resolved in these pages. The complexities of conceptual syntheses, however, are always encapsulated in a continuing process of contemplation, speculation, and reconciliation of experimental designs. These complexities are pointed to by a few of the authors, but less in a manner that provokes resolution of problems than one that stimulates discussion.

REFERENCE

Kuhn, T. S. (1970). *The Structure of Scientific Revolutions*. 2d ed. Chicago: University of Chicago Press.

ACKNOWLEDGMENTS

In June 1986 The Brunswick Institute sponsored a seminar at the Columbia Club of New York on the current status of multidisciplinary gerontology. It now seems clear to the editors, who participated in the seminar, that the inspiration for our present work derived directly from this meeting. We therefore wish to thank others at the seminar for their contributions: Guido Celano, Sara Harris, and Joseph P. Pedoto, all of whom, in both clinical and theoretical aspect, are part of the growing collectivity of those who engage in gerontological studies.

Our thanks go as well to Loomis Mayer and the editorial staff at Greenwood Press for facilitating the production of this volume. Our families have been most supportive in the face of the time devoted to this project. Our special thanks, then, to Ray Jordan and Cressida Osgood, and to Howard and David Sontz.

The Science
and
Practice of
Gerontology

1. INTRODUCTION. WITHIN AND BEYOND THE ACADEMY: BACKGROUNDS TO GERONTOLOGY RESEARCH AND PRACTICE

Ann H.L. Sontz

In E. V. Cowdry's classic, medically oriented volume, *The Care of the Geriatric Patient* (1958), various authors explore the status of the subspecialty of geriatrics as seen from the province of established disciplines in which this subspecialty has achieved substantial roots and recognition. The same approach is taken in this volume. This introductory chapter provides a brief background perspective to the chapters that follow by drawing together a few themes that appear within them, but that may warrant more elucidation than disciplinary reviews might want to provide. These themes are: (1) the growth of aging studies as measured by Ph.D. productivity, especially in the "core" fields of sociology, social work, and anthropology; (2) the nature of public and private grantmaking for gerontology research endeavors; and (3) clinical gerontology in light of legislative and private sector definition on the one hand, and the problems of health service intervention in a pluralistic society on the other.

In the process of the discussion I hope to have conveyed some sense of the opportunities and constraints in contemporary gerontology as viewed as a personal activity both within the academy and beyond our university systems.

CURRENTS IN DOCTORAL PRODUCTIVITY

The dramatic rise in the number of older adults in our population is amply documented in the pages that follow. Such demographic shifts have provoked policy studies, attitudinal and sociocultural research, a focus on age-linked illnesses, to mention a very few areas tied to an upsurge in scholarly activity. Indeed, gerontology instruction itself has increased significantly since the 1950s, and its dispersion among American campuses has evolved trenchantly as well (Peterson, 1986, 1987). The growth of gerontology as considered a subfield

Table 1.1
Gerontology Area Focus Ph.D.s in Anthropology, Sociology, Social Work, as a
Proportion of Disciplinary Ph.D.s, 1963–1985

Discipline	Total No. PhDs	Percent Gerontology PhDs
Anthropology	3,094	3.0%
Sociology	5,912	6.4%
Social Work	1,751	9.8%
Total	10,757	6.0%

Source: Derived from American Doctoral Dissertations' yearly
           catalogue, University Microfilms, Ann Arbor, Michigan.
           "Anthropology" as used here and in the text refers to
           cultural or social anthropology.

within a discipline or as a discipline in its own right has been a matter of some debate and discussion and is detailed by Wood, Parham, and Teitelman (Chapter 9) who present us with a rather thorough review of current feelings and ambivalences.

Researchers' enthusiasms have not, however, been dampened by such debates. A reading of the review articles by Birren and colleagues in the *Journal of Gerontology* from 1971 will indicate a substantial growth in Ph.D. production in a variety of disciplines, with a list of gerontology doctoral theses by author, topic, and university affiliation. For our present purposes, a brief overview of a subset of participants in this growth, namely doctoral production in aging studies within anthropology, sociology, and social work, may be illustrative of a few trends over the past decades or from 1963, when social work doctorates began registering in *American Doctoral Dissertations*, to 1985. Here, we will see an upswing in gerontology doctoral productivity in these fields, but the same encouraging development may be found in psychology and, to a smaller extent, in biology as well.

Table 1.1 indicates that gerontology doctorates as a total of all doctorates produced between 1963–1985 represented 3 percent in anthropology, 6.4 percent in sociology, and 9.8 percent in social work. Degree of gerontology penetration into disciplinary work may also be gauged by comparing aging studies Ph.D. productivity in earlier and more recent time periods (Table 1.2). In 1963–1967 anthropologists producing gerontology doctorates stood at only 6 percent of the total, but rose to 15 of all doctorates in that field between 1980–1985. Gerontology penetration of sociology doctoral work has remained similar throughout the years, but social work Ph.D.s with a focus on aging grew from 4 percent of the total in the early 1960s to 15 percent in the early 1980s.

Table 1.2
Gerontology Focus Ph.D.s as a Proportion of Disciplinary Ph.D.s by Time Segment, 1963–1985

	Anthropology	Sociology	Social Work
1963–1967	6%	33%	4%
1968–1973	13%	32%	6%
1974–1979	25%	29%	13%
1980–1985	15%	32%	15%

Source: Derived from American Doctoral Dissertations' yearly catalogue, University Microfilms, Ann Arbor, Michigan. "Anthropology" as used here and in the text refers to cultural or social anthropology.

One of the varied factors mediating gerontology focus Ph.D. growth on the disciplinary scene is that aging studies at the level of doctoral production have risen along with the numerical expansion of the elderly in our population. In social work there has been a concomitant tendency for the doctoral holder to be valued as an administrative figure and in the university professoriate. Tempered research funding, as outlined below, may have negated these academic energies somewhat, particularly the anthropological muse that appropriately thrives on research at distant points encompassing extensive travel costs and time duration. Lack of appropriate funds might therefore have negatively molded aging studies in that discipline, which saw a 10 percent decline in gerontology focus Ph.D. productivity since the heydays of the 1970s. Hornum and Glascock's (Chapter 5) well-argued discussion of the future of anthropological gerontology, however, indicates that ethnomethodological approaches have been able to bend fruitfully to communities close to home. Remaining elder studies in anthropology, moreover, present a multidisciplinary audience with no mere catalogue of exotica— but rather provide a basis for crosscultural considerations so necessary for emergent understandings of the universal processes of aging.

Against this backdrop of episodic rises and declines of Ph.D.s in the disciplines surveyed, the actual number of institutions of higher learning producing aging studies doctorates in those fields rose unimpeded (by 22 percent) from 1965–1985 (see Table 1.3). Table 1.4 shows a clustering of doctoral production in only sixteen university hands, however, and implies that an expansion of gerontology instruction has been nevertheless accompanied by a congregation of area Ph.D. productivity at a relatively few institutions. That fully 75 percent of all aging studies Ph.D.s in anthropology, sociology, and social work evinced a

Table 1.3
**Social Gerontology Ph.D. Producing Universities as a Proportion of All Doctoral
Producers, by Year**

Year	No. University PhD Producers	% Universities With Gerontology PhDs
1965	191	8 (4%)
1975	244	20 (8%)
1985	277	72 (26%)

Source: Derived from American Doctoral Dissertations' yearly
           catalogue, University Microfilms, Ann Arbor, Michigan.
           "Anthropology" as used here and in the text refers to
           cultural or social anthropology.

pattern of "scatteration" over hundreds of other institutions also pointed to a potentially healthy spread of research precedents upon which others seeking the advanced degree can build. Aging studies as a significant research enterprise began only in the 1960s. Its development, as measured in both predoctoral and postdoctoral work, is partially reflected in this book, which speaks to historical as well as contemporary relationships between scholarship and aging issues.

Numbers, of course, tell us little of dissertation quality; they simply chart growth patterns here taken as an indication that aging studies in certain critical fields have become attractive as a research activity at an early phase of academic productivity. Nor do these growth patterns provide us with a link between such an early phase and later work, so that we need further academic monitoring in order to clarify an assumed bond as well as an association of such personnel in present gerontology instructional units. We also need further research on the integration of gerontology focus Ph.D.s and postdoctoral researchers in graduate medical contexts, for there is a real need for multidisciplinary approaches and clinical applications even while geriatric training is still moving at a decidedly cautious pace (Sontz, 1986; see also Chapter 6 by Calkins and Karuza).

It is possible that niches for area focus gerontology researchers may come available as teaching positions in the increasing number of gerontology degree and certificate programs at both the graduate and undergraduate levels. Sociology, biology, and psychology appear with considerable frequency in undergraduate programs that offer a concentration, major, minor, or certificate in gerontology (Sullivan, 1985). Similar frequency patterns will be found at the master's level. There is as yet little evidence, however, that such academic positioning tied to disciplinary work, though in gerontology instruction units, is tied intimately to the understandings of aging studies.

Table 1.4
Selected Universities as Significant Social Gerontology Ph.D. Producers, 1963–1985

University*	No. PhDs	
		no. PhDs: 163
Brandeis	26	
Columbia	22	
Michigan	16	
Wisconsin (Madison)	12	
Southern California	9	
Case Western Reserve	9	
Berkeley	8	
Syracuse	8	
UCLA (S. Francisco)	8	
Northwestern	7	
Cornell	7	
Boston	7	
Arizona	6	
UCLA (L.A.)	6	
Utah	6	
Minnesota	6	

*Significant university producers are defined as those producing 1% or more of the total doctorates in aging studies with anthropology, sociology and social work between 1963-1985, or 646 doctorates.

Source: Derived from American Doctoral Dissertations' yearly catalogue, University Microfilms, Ann Arbor, Michigan. "Anthropology" as used here and in the text refers to cultural or social anthropology.

These and other clarifications linked to processes of academization also need to be further examined in light of manpower and training issues in the gerontology subspecialty. If, as Peterson (1987) has remarked, current gerontology instructional units are not leading to a Ph.D. or research track but rather are overwhelmingly oriented toward occupations in the broader labor market, then the supply of academic niches for the aging studies Ph.D. or postdoctoral researcher may show an appropriate gain. Of the many paradoxes that faced the academy in the postwar decades, one was a misconception of a faculty shortage in spite of a growing supply of Ph.D.s (McCaughey, 1984). In contrast, it is possible that the "gerontology collectivity" may face a rising need for doctoral-level instructors and researchers on an expanding number of campuses in the near future and an inability to keep close pace with this need because of shortfalls in appropriately trained personnel. These speculations must nevertheless be weighed against certain critical actualities: (1) varying factors have kept gerontology focus Ph.D.s at a small number despite growth in overall aging studies Ph.D. productivity; (2) fiscal restraints in research funding and in university budgets can limit postdoctoral aging studies work and negatively influence program growth and hiring practices; and (3) universities face declining student enrollments even in the face of increasing student interest in gerontology credentialing and coursework.

AN OVERVIEW OF GRANTMAKING FOR GERONTOLOGY

Issues surrounding academic gerontology raise questions about research funding, its origins, and trends. The National Institute on Aging (NIA) was founded only in 1974 as part of the National Institutes of Health (NIH). By 1985 the great majority of NIH monies were awarded to the medical schools, and the budget of the NIA tended to mirror a biomedical thrust though grants to social gerontology grew gradually (NIH, 1985). A focus on aging research and biomedicine has not really been tempered by the grantmaking practices of the philanthropic foundations. Data from 444 endowed funds with $1 million or more in assets indicate that only 2.8 percent devoted themselves to grantmaking for the elderly in 1985 (Nee and Bracco, 1986; Sontz, 1989).

To some extent, the Administration on Aging (AOA) has addressed questions concerning the bonds among family and the elderly, community, and ethnicity. These are issues that complement the NIA's Older People and Society and Total Behavioral Sciences funding agenda. Available information, from 1979–1981, indicates that university personnel received 58 percent of all AOA research grants, but 49 percent of these were dispersed in four areas only—California; Washington, D.C.; New York; and Pennsylvania. It seems therefore likely that federal funding concentrations broadly reflect the tendency for Ph.D. productivity in aging studies to cluster in a relatively few institutional hands. Indeed, generic funding for science on the part of federal agencies continues to focus primarily on 50 prominent universities out of more than 200, among them the significant aging studies Ph.D. producers (Sommer, 1987). Moreover, NIA monies, as do general federal monies, highly favor health and basic research in the life sciences (ibid.). In this pattern may inhere the medicalization of aging research as well as the fact that much of the creative work in sociocultural and psychogerontology discussed in this volume was conceived and concluded in an environment hedged round with shrunken fiscal supports. It is highly probable that there will continue to be a gerontology research dependence on governmental funding both for predoctoral and postdoctoral endeavors. With the exception of some limited biomedical subventions, this dependence is not being loosened by current activities surrounding foundation largesse. Diversified supports emanating from the government to nonbiomedical aging studies as well as a growth of foundation accessibility to social and psychogerontology researchers would be a welcome addition to the grantmaking scene and would conjoin with a growing movement of nonbiomedical scholars into a rapidly expanding academic field.

COMMENTARY ON CLINICAL GERONTOLOGY

The reader will find that practice settings for the clinician are many and varied and range from counseling to geriatric medicine, and from social work practice to geriatric rehabilitation tied to normal aging processes and to functional declines (see Chapter 6 by Calkins and Karuza; Chapter 7 by Kalosieh and Pedoto; and Chapter 8 by Lowy). Practice settings encompass home, nursing setting, office, adult day center, hospital, and clinic. Legislative activity producing policies such as Medicare has spurred professional responses while it is also possible that the small but influential emphasis on foundation programming for the elderly has begun to create a limited but enriched vessel for the growth of practice niches as well. In the concluding chapter, Wood, Parham, and Teitelman integrate several facets of the growth of aging studies into a discussion of the beginnings of gerontology education, one trend of which is preparation for the labor market and the clinical fields.

A review of the chapters in the "practice" section will no doubt yield that no one practice model adequately factors in the complexities of health intervention with the frail elderly. Rather, two models seem to prevail. One of these assumes that the elderly individual is not an isolate, but rather is enmeshed, to a greater or lesser extent, in a rich psychosocial and cultural field that influences the character of illness onset and therapeutic planning. Human development studies have provided the basis for another model which argues that the life span can be analytically segmented into characteristic sequences, each of which, as in youth or late age, is marked by its own recognizable traits or criteria. What conditions, the biologist Edward Masoro asks, are merely associated with age or are dependent upon its presence? What distinctions among age groups, inquire the psychologists Hoyer and Hooker, can be anticipated in practice situations relative to cognitive abilities, psychomotor performance, or neuropathology? Or, then, are distinctions observed not coincident with late age at all, but best seen in light of intraindividual and interindividual differences? Practice, it is clear, especially in the hands of a sensitive and intuitive professional, tends to temper broad theories; yet what is universal to late age, what is subject to cultural definition, and what is an idiosyncratic reaction to aging remain essential background understandings that infuse practice decisions today.

Despite growth in practice niches and model development, there are few specific mandates as to the actual *social organization of service delivery* itself. The need for transdisciplinary efforts has been duly noted by Calkins and Karuza, but they still conclude that the multidisciplinary team often forms a type of ad hoc coalition rather than a structured and regularized affair. Academic territoriality may here be less important than limitations on practice privileges that militate against the expansion of a multidisciplinary team approach. A need for more interdisciplinary education within the gerontology enterprise is not here compromised. Multidisciplinary efforts require a sensitivity to others' intellectuality and mental categories; the absence of a team encircling the lone practitioner more than heightens the desirability of such sensitivities during the course of client evaluation and treatment scheduling. In this regard, the medical anthropologist with a gerontology background has often been underreported in the multidisciplinary team largely because of a sometimes consultative rather than direct practice role. Yet Hornum and Glascock's review of anthropological gerontology and their appended bibliography indicate strongly that a biologistic framework of practice can fruitfully be complemented by one that draws on variations in health behaviors according to cultural organization and specificity (see also Fabrega, 1971). Culturological, or even psychosocial, assumptions have far to go before they incisively penetrate clinical settings. This multidisciplinary guide, hopefully convenient in format, invites the practitioner to transcend disciplinary turfs where he or she will, at the same time, gain a sense of distinct disciplinary-based theoretical and clinical pathways. Despite constraints, aging studies are today a growing field for research and practice alike, and clinical gerontologists are in an admirable position to establish innovative liaisons between the two. Moreover, clinical as well as research activities are not static, but processual in nature. By evaluating and reevaluating the character of psychosocial, biological, and cultural factors influencing the health and well-being of elderly individuals, clinicians contribute to a crossfertilization of gerontological knowledge and thus make practice a creative and equal partner with theories of aging and related policy developments.

CONCLUSION

I believe that there exist two broad themes within this volume that can provide a guide to readers as they confront the rich detail that is now characteristic of a very healthy field with growing research and applied aspects. One is that there is an increased sense of parity among professionals within the gerontology enterprise. Both academicians and clinicians are increasingly perceived as interdependent within a professionalizing structure that is not necessarily hierarchical in nature. Certainly, one can no longer really question the desire for multidisciplinary sharing mechanisms in aging studies, only the manner in which these shall be evolved, organized, and applied.

Another theme, bearing on the multidisciplinary, and more of a background setting for academic discussions in this guide (Chapter 9) than a featured player, nevertheless bears being brought to consciousness wherever it may be thought that aging studies constitutes its own isolate within the academy at least insofar as its struggles for accreditation, standardization, departmentalization, and other key aspects of discipline-building are concerned. For example, "international" and "women's" studies are multidisciplinary subfields that continue to reflect strong disciplinary currents despite some departmental activity, academic programming, and university research centers. Similarly, the growth of these area studies has been wedded to critical trends underlying professionalization, though not in the clinical sense, variable funding supports, and intellectual reactivity in mediating environmental factors including demographic shifts. While insularity in multidisciplinary aging studies needs to be overcome, some thought might also be given to expanding the research gerontology enterprise to include the rich texture of these already existent subspecialties where overlaps of interest and approach may occur. Women's studies research centers, such as The Equity Policy Center and the Program of Policy Research on Women and Families, can prove valuable research aids for the purpose of clarifying the condition of older women in society. Data and understandings from international studies can constitute a fruitful program for gerontology research in comparative legislation and conditions governing late age adjustments across an extensive macrosocial reach. Shanas' earlier volume (Shanas et al., 1968) focusing on the status of older adults in the United States and Europe needs to be complemented by work from Southeast Asia, African nations, and the Middle East where international studies materials would enrich the aging studies repertoire with crossnational and progressive findings. All this goes into saying that subspecialization within the gerontology collectivity, or even what Wood, Parham, Teitelman, and others feel is an inevitable movement toward actual disciplinary specialization in the future, does not necessarily imply a coming parochialization as well. Indeed, aging studies appear anything but parochial, divided as they are into linked research and clinical components in varying organizational contexts. The separation of this volume into two sections, the one reflective largely of academic energies, the other of the rigors of diverse practice niches. acknowledges these different professional outlets. At the same time, the chapters present a variety of views as to how this current duality can best be actively related for the enhancement of aging studies in its current status as a subfield and for the betterment of our growing older adult population.

REFERENCES

Administration on Aging (1982). *Grants to Research on Aging, 1979–1981*.

Cowdry, E. V. (Ed.) (1958). *The Care of the Geriatric Patient*. St. Louis: C. V. Mosby.

Fabrega, H. (1971). Medical anthropology. In B. Siegel (Ed.), *Biennial Review of Anthropology*. Stanford, Calif.: Stanford University Press.

McCaughey, R. (1984). *International Studies and Academic Enterprise*. New York: Columbia University Press.

National Institutes of Health (1985). *The Search for Health*. Bethesda, Md.: NIH.

Nee, D. M., and Bracco, D. E. (1986). *Grantmaking for the Elderly*. New York: Florence V. Burden Foundation.

Peterson, D. A. (1986). *Extent of Gerontology Instruction in American Institutions of Higher Learning*. University of Southern California, at Los Angeles. Andrus Gerontology Center.

Peterson, D. A. (1987). *Gerontology Credentials*. University of Southern California, at Los Angeles. Andrus Gerontology Center.

Shanas, E. et al. (1968). *Old People in Three Industrial Societies*. New York: Atherton Press.

Sommer, J. (1987). Mapping federal funding. *American Scientist*, 75, 447–48.

Sontz, A.H.L. (1986). *Medical Education and Gerontology*. New Brunswick, N.J.: The Brunswick Institute on Aging.

Sontz, A.H.L. (1989). *Philanthropy and Gerontology: The Role of American Foundations*. Westport, Conn.: Greenwood Press.

Sullivan, E. N. (Ed.) (1985). *National Directory of Educational Programs in Gerontology*. 3d ed. Washington, D.C.: Association for Gerontology in Higher Education.

Part I
SCIENCE IN
GERONTOLOGY

2. THE BIOLOGY OF AGING

Edward J. Masoro

In basic biological terms, what is aging? The answer is that we do not know. This statement may be hard to accept because intuitively we feel we have an understanding of aging. We feel this way because we have no problem in distinguishing old animals and people from the young. However, this ease of distinction is based on observable or phenotypic characteristics associated with aging and not on knowledge of the fundamental biological processes involved.

This lack of knowledge is emphasized by the fact that most gerontologists have defined aging in terms of the decreasing ability of an organism to survive (Strehler, 1977). Indeed, after maturity has been reached the probability of dying increases with increasing age (Kohn, 1978). Although aging is clearly an important factor influencing mortality, many other factors can also be involved. Thus, a definition of aging based on mortality suffers from the fact that mortality is not a specific marker of aging; moreover, even if it were, mortality data provide little understanding of the basic processes involved.

CURRENT STATUS OF FACTUAL KNOWLEDGE

Many of the facts that were believed to be known about aging have either been disproven or require qualification because of recent research. An assessment of the current status of this factual knowledge base is therefore warranted.

In 1825, Gompertz, an English actuary, reported that in humans after maturity, the rate and probability of dying increase exponentially with increasing age (see Kohn, 1978). This has subsequently been found to be true of many animal species (Sacher, 1977). In considering the influence of age on mortality, the concept of age-specific death rate is defined as the number of individuals that have died during an age interval divided by the number of individuals alive during that age interval. After maturity, the age-specific death rate doubles at regular intervals; e.g., in the house mouse at 220-day intervals, in the beagle dog at 812-day intervals, and in the human American female as of 1969 at 3,100-day intervals (ibid).

Another mortality characteristic commonly discussed in relation to aging is life expectancy. *Life expectancy is defined as the mean length of life remaining for a population of a given age.* When birth is the age of reference, life expectancy is synonymous with the mean length of life of a population. Much is made of the fact that the life expectancy from birth of Americans (as well as that of the populations of most developed nations) has markedly increased during the twentieth century from about forty-seven years in 1900 to seventy-three years in 1980 (Fries and Crapo, 1981). Although this is clearly impressive, its importance in regard to aging is often exaggerated. Indeed, the protection of any animal species from environmental hazards that result in premature death will increase life expectancy (Kirkwood and Holliday, 1979). This does not imply that this protection has influenced the aging processes. Rather, the appropriate interpretation would seem to be that protection from environmental hazards by technological advances such as sanitation engineering, immunization, and antibiotics has permitted the population to age. Thus, the increase in life expectancy in the developed nations that has occurred during the twentieth century does not imply that the aging processes have been influenced but rather that a large population of aged people has been generated by the prevention of premature death. The impact of this demographic change on our society, of course, is great and focuses thought on both the aging processes and on the societal problems associated with a large fraction of the population being of advanced age.

The life span of a species, often referred to as the maximum life span, is the length of life of the longest-lived members of that species. The maximum life span, which is a characteristic of each species, is about one hundred years or so for humans, seventy years for elephants, twenty years for dogs, and three years for the house mouse (Kirkwood, 1985). The extension of the life span of a species would strongly indicate that the aging processes have been slowed. The life span of Americans during the twentieth century has remained at approximately one hundred years (Fries and Crapo, 1981), which indicates that the technological and medical advances of this century have not significantly influenced the aging processes.

The view that the life span can be extended has become popular in the lay literature. Nutritional and pharmacologic agents and life-style changes have been promoted in this regard (Schneider and Reed, 1985). In many cases, a distinction has not been made between life expectancy and life span. When such a distinction is made it is clear that only one manipulation has been shown to reproducibly extend the life span of a mammalian species and that manipulation is food restriction in rodents (Masoro, 1985). In addition to increasing life span and life expectancy, food restriction retards most, but not all, age-related physiological changes as well as most age-related disease processes (Maeda et al., 1985). It is not known whether food restriction would have similar actions in mammalian species other than rodents. The relevant research has not been done because of the great cost in money and other resources that would be required to execute such a study in species with life spans greater than those of rats, hamsters, and mice. Moreover, it is not likely that many would adopt a lifelong food restriction regimen even if it were found to be effective in humans. However, research on food restriction in rodents is of importance to humans because uncovering the mechanisms by which food restriction retards the aging processes may well provide the database needed for the development of effective interventions of human aging.

The fact that the life span of mammalian species varies markedly even though all species age in what appears to be a qualitatively similar fashion has led most biologists to feel that genetics play a major role in aging (Masoro, 1987a). This view is supported by the fact that in humans the mean difference in longevity between fraternal twins was found to be twice as great as that in identical twins (Kallman and Jarvik, 1959). Also, Goodrick (1975) estimated from a study of inbred mouse strains that half of the variance associated with longevity was due to genetic factors. Although there is general agreement that genetics plays an important role in aging, the nature of the genetic event remains to be defined. Indeed, whether a few genes are involved or several thousand genes is subject to debate (Kirkwood, 1985).

It is generally believed that physiological deterioration is a characteristic of aging (Masoro, 1986). Much of the basis for this belief comes from the pioneering work of the laboratory of Nathan Shock (Brandfonbrener et al., 1955; Davies and Shock, 1950; Shock and Yiengst, 1950; Shock and Yiengst, 1955). Although this physiological deterioration can readily be demonstrated in studies that examine unscreened populations cross-sectionally, recent research indicates that much of this physiological deterioration may be due to coexisting disease or life-style rather than to aging per se.

For example, casual observation has led to the generally held belief that functional deterioration of the nervous system is a hallmark of aging. This impression appears to be based on observing the performance of individuals with age-associated diseases such as Alzheimer's disease. In the apparent absence of such a disease, however, there are changes in nervous system function with advanced age but they are not marked and involve a mild loss of memory, a somewhat reduced ability to learn new tasks, and a decrease in the speed of processing by brain (Katzman, 1985). Indeed, longitudinal studies show that most brain functions considered to represent intelligence remain essentially intact throughout life (Katzman and Terry, 1983). Moreover, the slow reaction time that characterizes the aged is in part a result of life-style since increasing physical activity of old people speeds up their reaction time (Spirduso, 1974).

Clearly, it is difficult to know to what extent physiological deterioration observed in old people and animals is due to aging per se and to what extent it is secondary to disease or life-style. A major research challenge is the design of studies that can sort out the contribution of aging as a distinct variable to the physiological and psychosocial changes observed with advancing age.

Some diseases are age-associated; i.e., they are more prevalent at advanced ages or in a specific age range (Upton, 1977). The extent to which these diseases are a part of or secondary to aging processes cannot be answered with our current knowledge base. For example, clinical manifestations of atherosclerosis such as myocardial infarction and stroke are increasingly prevalent at advanced ages. However, atherosclerosis begins at a young age (Lakatta, 1985) and progresses in severity with time. In regard to the relationship of atherosclerosis to aging, there are the following possibilities: (1) both share the same time frame but are related in no other way; (2) atherogenesis is promoted by the aging processes; (3) atherogenesis is part of the aging processes. The current available database does not enable a choice to be made between these possibilities (Bates and Gangloff, 1987).

Another example is Alzheimer's disease which becomes increasingly common after forty years of age (Katzman, 1985). Morphologically the disease is characterized by neurofibrillary tangles and neuritic plaques in brain areas. Unlike atherosclerosis, there is no morphologic evidence for the progression of Alzheimer's disease from a young age. Nevertheless, such progression may be occurring at a biochemical rather than morphologic level. However, another possibility is that the biological environment of an old individual is required for the occurrence and progression of Alzheimer's disease. Again, the currently available database does not permit a choice between these possibilities.

In an attempt to provide further understanding of the relationship between aging and age-associated disease, Brody and Schneider (1986) have developed a view of age-associated diseases in which they are classified as either age-dependent or age-related. *Age-dependent diseases* are defined as those diseases in which the pathogenesis appears to involve the normal aging processes. *Age-related diseases* are defined as those diseases that have a temporal relationship to the host but are not necessarily related to the aging processes. Examples that the authors give for age-dependent diseases are coronary heart disease, cerebrovascular diseases, Type II diabetes, osteoporosis, Alzheimer's disease, and Parkinson's disease. In regard to age-related diseases, the authors cite the following: multiple sclerosis, amyotrophic lateral sclerosis, and most but not all cancers. The major support for this classification is that age-dependent diseases increase exponentially with increasing age in tandem with the age-specific death rate and that age-related diseases, while showing an association with a particular age range, do not increase exponentially with increasing age over the life span. Although this hypothesis and classification are intriguing, the database upon which they are supported is weak.

Unfortunately, it is difficult to obtain clear evidence that aging plays a pathogenic role in an age-associated disease; so difficult that as of now there is not such evidence for any disease. Masoro (1987b) described a way of obtaining such evidence for chronic nephropathy in rats, a major age-associated disease of this species, and also suggested a possible way of doing so for human atherosclerosis. Since space does not permit a presentation of these experimental approaches, the interested reader is referred to the above cited reference.

CURRENT TRENDS IN RESEARCH ON AGING

Research Based on Genetics

As discussed earlier, aging appears to have a strong genetic component. There is much current work in this area such as the research on the human genetic diseases that have a number of features that resemble premature aging (Brown, 1985). Examples are: Progeria characterized by balding, loss of subcutaneous tissue, aged appearance of skin, and median age of death of twelve years; Werner's Syndrome characterized by premature whiting and graying of hair and cataract formation, aged appearance of skin, loss of muscle mass, and death in the fourth decade of life; and Down's Syndrome characterized by premature graying of hair and baldness, cataracts, and death before forty years of age. Another area that has been active recently is that of gene expression and aging (Richardson et al., 1985). For instance, it has been found that the levels of mRNA species coding for aldolase, PEP-carboxykinase, pyruvate kinase, phenylalanine hydroxylase, ornithine transcarbamylase, and arginosuccinate synthetase decrease with age. Indeed, a broad spectrum of research is being initiated on the genetics of aging using the tools of molecular biology.

Research Based on Free Radical Theory

The free radical theory of aging first proposed in 1954 by Denon Harman currently has many proponents (Harman, 1981). Free radicals are chemical substances that have electronic structures that make them very highly reactive. They are continuously generated by the action of ionizing radiation and a variety of other nonenzymatic and enzymatic reactions both within cells and in the extracellular compartments of mammalian organisms. However, the most important source is oxygen free radical generation during the consumption of oxygen by mitochondria of the cells (Nohl and Hegner, 1978). Free radicals can cause a spectrum of cellular damage including oxidative alterations of long-lived molecules (e.g., DNA, collagen), oxidative degradation of mucopolysaccharides, generation of lipofuscin, and alterations of biological membranes (Harman, 1981). However, cells have many defense mechanisms protecting them from free radical damage (e.g., antioxidants such as tocopherols and carotenes and protective enzymes such as peroxidases and superoxide dismutase). The cell is also able to repair damaged molecules and cellular structures. Research strategies are now being used to study the role of free radicals in the aging processes. For instance, in our laboratory, the effects of food restriction regimens that retard the aging processes are being explored in regard to their effect on free radical formation, free radical protective mechanisms, and free radical damage.

Research Based on Hayflick Phenomenon

Hayflick and Moorhead (1961) showed that human fibroblast-like cells in culture have a limited period of active proliferation. Subsequent work suggested that this limited *in vitro* proliferative potential is determined by the number of cell divisions that have occurred rather than by calendar time in culture. Hayflick and Moorhead proposed that this loss of growth potential is an intrinsic property of euploid somatic cells and that this type of *in vitro* system may be an appropriate model for the investigation of some aspects of aging at the cellular level. If so, simplicity of the system makes it a most attractive one for investigating basic aging processes. Unfortunately, the validity of this system as a model for exploring the aging processes occurring in the intact organism is still a subject of controversy (Norwood and Smith, 1985), and much effort is being made to learn whether or not it is a valid model. This involves studying cellular functions other than proliferative activity, which requires the cultivation of different cell types, and the extension of the cell culture studies to animal models such as rodents thus enabling penetrating studies relating *in vivo* aging to that occurring in cell culture systems.

Research Based on Food Restriction Phenomenon

As discussed earlier, food restriction in rodents is the only manipulation that has clearly been shown to retard the aging processes in mammals (Masoro, 1985). The major basis for this claim is the extension of life span, but further support comes from the retardation of most age-associated physiological change and the prevention or retardation of most age-associated disease by food restriction. Learning the mechanisms by which food restriction retards the aging processes should provide considerable insight on the nature of basic aging processes as well as a database for developing effective interventions of human aging. Currently much as yet unpublished research is ongoing and is aimed at understanding the mechanisms by which food restriction influences the aging processes.

Research on Biomarkers of Aging

A biomarker of aging is a biological event or measurement that can estimate or predict one or more of the aging processes. The great current interest in biomarkers of aging is their potential role in guiding research on aging, in assessing the effects of pharmacologic and environment agents on aging, and in evaluating the biological age of an individual in relation to the ability of the individual to carry out a given kind of work (e.g., functioning as a railroad worker, a physician, a construction worker, etc.). At this time, there are no generally agreed upon biomarkers of aging (Reff and Schneider, 1982).

Part of the confusion about biomarkers of aging is that this general term is applied when referring to very different uses. Indeed, these uses can be classified as follows: (1) the estimation of chronologic age; (2) the estimation of biological age; (3) the prediction of the occurrence of an age-associated disease; (4) the prediction of the impending death of an individual; (5) the prediction of the life span of a species and the influence of a manipulation on that life span.

There is a good marker for estimating chronologic age and that is amino acid racemization in structural proteins sequestered from metabolic turnover (Bada and Brown, 1980). This use of a biomarker is of value only when knowledge of the age of an animal or person is desired for whom the birth date is not known.

Biomarkers that estimate biological age would, of course, be of great value to researchers as well as to the decisions that must be made in regard to matters such as retirement. The questions that must be answered are (1) Is there such a thing as biological age distinct from chronologic age? and (2) If so, can biological age be assessed? A major problem that arises in addressing these questions is the fact that different systems in the same individual can age independently (e.g., the occurrence of grayness of the hair does not correlate with the development of deafness) and the fact that the rate of an aging of an individual is not constant during sequential intervals of the life span (Costa and McCrae, 1980). Investigators have recognized the inappropriateness of assessing biological age on the basis of a single process and have turned to examining several systems simultaneously. The results have been analyzed by multiple regression analysis and by "profile" analysis. As of now, the evidence indicates that these analyses provide no better information about biological age than does chronologic age (Costa and McCrae, 1985).

There are biomarkers that predict the occurrence of age-associated diseases; they are usually referred to as risk factors for that disease. Examples are: arterial blood pressure as a risk factor for stroke (Kannel, 1985), and the serum concentration of low-density lipoprotein cholesterol as a risk factor for coronary heart disease (Schoenfeld, 1984). It is not clear that these risk factors provide information on aging because the relationship of these diseases to the aging process remains to be defined.

Predictors of impending death are considered by many to be biomarkers of aging. Impairment of pulmonary function is an example of such a predictor (Beaty et al., 1982). Surprisingly, cardiovascular disease and cancer rather than pulmonary disease are major causes of these deaths. However, the impairment of pulmonary function, which clearly appears to be a predictor of cardiovascular disease and cancer, may or may not be a marker of aging. As discussed earlier, mortality data may provide little information about aging. Thus, predictors of mortality in the absence of other evidence cannot be viewed as biomarkers of aging.

Predictors of the life span of a species have the potential of being valid biomarkers of aging. Indeed, it is likely that a manipulation that increases the life span of a species does so by retarding the aging processes. Thus, physiological events that are also influenced by that manipulation might well be valid markers of the aging processes. Unfortunately, as discussed earlier, only food restriction has been shown to increase the life span of a mammalian species. It is impossible to know if the influence on a physiological process by food restriction is due to the retardation of the aging processes or to some other action of food restriction. To address this problem will require the extension of the life span of a mammalian species by more than one manipulation. If several manipulations that extend the life span of a species modulated a particular physiological process in the same manner, it would be highly likely that the particular physiological process is a valid biomarker of aging. Of course, the development of such manipulations is a sizable challenge. Clearly, much remains to be done on the development of biomarkers of aging, and research in this field is being and will be vigorously pursued.

HISTORICAL ROOTS

This review of the current status of knowledge and research activities in the biology of aging suggests that biological gerontology is far less advanced than most areas of biology. To understand the reasons for this requires a consideration of the historical roots of biological gerontology as a subfield.

Over the ages, the great thinkers have been concerned with aging. In his writings, Aristotle contemplated the fact that different species have defined life spans that differ markedly from each other and also noted the functional deterioration with age, in particular the loss of reproductive function and the changes in nervous system function (Griffin, 1950). Leonardo da Vinci made careful morphologic assessments of human aging and on the basis of these observations concluded that vascular changes underlie aging (Belt, 1952). In 1623, *Historia Vitae et Mortis,* authored by Sir Francis Bacon, appeared. In this work Bacon presents his concept of the vital spirit and discusses how it is influenced by life process resulting in mortality (Strong, 1952).

Unfortunately, over the ages, many who made pronouncements about aging were not thoughtful people. For instance, the European alchemists sought or claimed to have found "the elixer of life," a preparation purported to extend life (Comfort, 1979). Even today this kind of thinking continues in the claims that particular life-styles (such as specific dietary and exercise regimens) will extend life despite the absence of valid evidence. The unsubstantiated claims and the people who make them have associated the field of aging studies with unscientific endeavors and have deterred serious, able scientists from engaging in aging research.

Of course, there have been scientists of towering stature who have addressed the issue of aging. Examples are Szilard (1959) who proposed a stochastic model of aging and Burnet (1970) who developed an immunologic theory. Unfortunately, aging was only a minor interest of these distinguished scientists, and experimental follow-through providing adequate testing of these theories did not occur. Indeed, a major problem has been the fact that many of the scientists who have proposed theories of aging have not been concerned with the experimental testing of them, resulting in a field that is cluttered with untestable theories.

It is a fact that until recently most experimental biologists have shied away from aging research. However, the negative connotation of the field is by no means the only reason for this. Another major reason is the direction biology has taken in recent years along with the contemporary training of biologists, which have been focused on detailed molecular events with little emphasis on global processes. This has resulted in the neglect of broad integrative biology and in experimentalists incapable of addressing complex problems such as aging. Another reason is a form of intellectual snobbery that has pervaded biology, which focuses on learning mechanism (preferably molecular mechanism) and shuns all descriptive studies even when (as is the case with biological gerontology) such data are essential for the progress of the field. Finally, the need for young faculty to publish quickly and often to survive in academic institutions makes them unwilling to execute the long-term research often required in gerontology.

Since 1950, however, a few investigators have explored aging in a careful, logical fashion. An outstanding example is Nathan Shock, who systematically collected fundamental data so necessary for the further study of aging. In a paper (Lang and Richie, 1986) written by two former students in honor of his eightieth birthday it was pointed out that not only did Dr. Shock develop the approaches needed for the exploration of aging but also trained those who have played and will play a major role in the study of the biology of aging during the last half of the twentieth century and on into the twenty-first century.

Institutional factors have also mediated the development of aging studies in biology. With the creation in 1974 of the National Institute on Aging as one of the National Institutes of Health a major influence on aging research in the United States began. The availability of grant support from this institute earmarked for aging led immediately to the development of aging research proposals from many investigators. Unfortunately, many successful proposals were poorly designed because of the lack of understanding of aging research by the scientists applying and by the peer review group evaluating the proposals. The investigators, often experts in a particular biological field, explored the effects of aging in their area of biological expertise without formulating important gerontological questions, using appropriate animal models, showing concerns for the availability of life table data, disease and nutritional status of the animals, and a host of other factors. The NIH peer review system was developed so as to assess particular biological disciplines, but aging was not one of them. The result was that often no one reviewing the proposal had any understanding of aging research. With time this situation has gradually been rectified. An increasing number of investigators have become knowledgeable about aging research; the National Institute on Aging has developed review committees with great knowledge of aging research and, increasingly, other peer review groups either have members with such knowledge or seek consultations with scientists who do.

FUTURE NEEDS

The rapid development of any area of biology requires hypotheses that can be tested experimentally. Biogerontology is no exception. As discussed earlier, many of the theories of aging were developed with little concern about the experimental testing of their validity. For example, the Free Radical Theory of Aging has many proponents and much data are consistent with it. What is needed now are studies that test the causal relationship of free radicals to the aging processes. The challenge to the biological gerontologist is to design such experiments. Another popular theory of aging is the Immune Theory. Although immune deficiencies and autoimmunity occur with aging (Hausman and Weksler, 1985), whether these immune changes are the result of primary aging processes or are causally related to aging has yet to be defined. Clearly, therefore, major needs of biological gerontology are (1) the development of theories of aging that can be experimentally tested, and (2) experimental designs for the testing of existing theories.

The evidence that genes play a major role in aging (Masoro, 1987a) mandates that emphasis in future research be placed on the genetics of aging. This should include identifying the genes that are involved in the aging processes. Particular emphasis should be placed on regulatory genes since the evidence points to their playing a major role. Mechanisms should be explored that can cause modification in gene structure with age such as intrinsic mutagenesis, loss of fidelity of the protein biosynthesis machinery, crosslinking of DNA, genetic amplifications and deletions, and slow virus action. Mechanisms should also be explored that modify gene expression such as codon restriction, neuroendocrine modifications, progressive transcriptional repression, and allelic exclusion.

Another area that requires development is that of model systems for the study of aging. Cell culture systems (often called *in vitro* aging) are attractive because they provide ease of experimental manipulations, the ability to rapidly explore specific questions and potentially circumvent the need to use aging animals. As stated earlier, the validity of these cell culture systems as models for the study of aging processes that occur in the intact animal has not been established. Significant future effort should address this issue since, if cell culture systems can be shown to provide a valid model for the study of aging, progress in aging research is likely to markedly increase.

Animals, particularly those with short life spans, such as rats and mice, are currently the most important models for the study of aging and they are likely to continue to be in the immediate future. Indeed, even to validate or invalidate the cell culture system as a model will require the use of animal models. There is great need to further develop animal models for specific areas of research. However, an even more important issue for the scientific community to address is the hindrance to use of animal models posed by the animal rights groups and related concerned organizations. As a biological gerontologist who utilizes animal models, I can personally attest to the fact that the response of government agencies and university administrators to the animal rights movement has often involved inappropriate harassment of investigators rather than carefully thought-out constructive responses. Certainly, humane treatment of animal models is a must. Indeed, animal models for aging research require uniquely excellent care. For instance, the rats used in our laboratory are protected from any exposure to pathogenic organisms, are provided a constant, defined environment including temperature control, controlled turnover of air, humidity control, defined diet with optimal levels of specific nutrients, and many other procedures aimed at eliminating environmental hazards. Unfortunately, it seems that animal rights groups are more interested in no use of animal models than careful, humane use.

In responding to the pressures from such groups, it must be recognized that the use of animal models for aging research is essential if we are going to gain a basic understanding of the aging processes in the foreseeable future. Moreover, it also must be recognized that such knowledge is essential for developing the interventions of the detrimental aspects of aging needed to meet the demographic challenge of the twenty-first century. This message must be brought forcefully to the attention of the administrators of universities and government agencies. It is also important that federal and state legislators recognize that it is not enough to provide the financial resources for biomedical studies of aging but that the laws of the land must promote and certainly not hinder the use of animal models. *The concept that mathematical models and computer technology can replace animal models in uncovering the nature of the aging processes must also be clearly shown not to be valid to those who are not biological scientists.* By this I do not aim to deny the important role that mathematical models and computer technology can play in biogerontology but rather to make it clear that they do not replace animal models. Their importance resides in the powerful tools they provide for the design and analysis of animal model research.

It is clear that valid biomarkers of aging in animal models and human subjects are sorely needed if rapid progress in biogerontology is to occur. It is also clear that at this time no such markers have been validated; and, as discussed earlier, to do so is most difficult to accomplish. However, so important are valid bio-markers that much future effort must be made in developing approaches for the validating of biomarkers of aging.

Approaches aimed at attaining life span extension will also be the focus of future research. In part, the reason for this will be the same as it was for the alchemists of previous centuries, basically the desire of some people for im-mortality or, in lieu of that, a very long life. However, in addition to that human desire, there are compelling scientific reasons to explore life span extension manipulations via animal models. Such manipulations provide an important approach to learning about the aging process, as was discussed in the section on food restriction. In addition, different manipulations that extend the life span of an animal model may provide the best approach to the validating of biomarkers of aging.

Although most of us have human aging as our primary interest, the human subject has proven to be a difficult model to use for the study of the biology of aging. The major reasons for this are: (1) the fact that it is difficult to carry out meaningful longitudinal studies in such a long-lived species and thus the heavy reliance on cross-sectional studies, and (2) the problem of obtaining control of and even full knowledge of the lifelong environment including the life-style of the subject. Ways of addressing these issues are beginning to emerge and further development of these approaches is necessary for the meaningful study of aging human subjects. A few of these problems and emerging approaches warrant discussion.

The issue of disease, which was not considered in many of the early cross-sectional human studies in regard to age-associated physiological or behavioral change, is addressed in most recent work. Indeed, the Baltimore Longitudinal Study of Aging has focused on what is called normative aging, in which the subjects are screened to assure that discernable disease is absent. A particularly striking example is the cross-sectional study of Garry et al. (1982) who limited their research on nutritional status of the aged to subjects with no known medical illnesses and no prescription medication. These elderly subjects were found to have a nutritional status similar to the young. Two problems emerge from such studies. How small a fraction of the total population of a particular age group does such a select population represent? Since this question was not addressed in the Garry et al. study, it is not clear how useful this information will be to the practitioner. More important theoretically is the assumption that age-associated diseases have nothing to do with normal aging processes. Clearly, future research on humans must address these issues.

Longitudinal studies have been done with human populations and, relative to the findings of earlier cross-sectional studies, some of the results are surprising. An excellent example is the longitudinal study of Lindeman et al. (1985) on 254 subjects of the Baltimore Longitudinal Study of Aging who appeared to be free of renal or urinary tract disease and were not receiving diuretic or antihypertensive therapy. Cross-sectional studies (Goldman, 1977) have clearly shown that glomerular filtration rate falls with age. In this longitudinal study the subjects ranged in age from thirty to ninety years and their glomerular filtration rates were measured over long periods of time (up to twenty-four years). About two-thirds of these subjects showed an age-associated fall in glomerular filtration rate similar to that reported in previous cross-sectional studies. However, one-third of the subjects did not show a decrease in glomerular filtration rate with age. Much further work of this type must be done since it showed that a physiological deterioration that was felt to be an inevitable consequence of aging does not necessarily occur.

This general issue was recently addressed by Rowe and Kahn (1987). They point out that aging research has focused on the mean level of physiological and behavioral parameters of various age groups, and in the absence of disease the conclusion has been that the change in those mean levels indicates a loss of function due to the aging processes. They note there is substantial heterogeneity within age groups and a significant number at advanced ages do not show this loss in function. They suggest that the subjects in the normal aging population (i.e., people free of disease) should be classified in two categories: one is the usual aging group that shows functional loss; the other is the successful aging group that does not show such a loss. They further postulate that the losses in function in the usual aging group may not relate to the aging processes per se but may be secondary to diet, exercise, personal habit, and psychosocial factors and, therefore, that functional loss due to aging processes per se has been overstated. These are important concepts and should be the focus of much future research aimed at determining the validity of this view. Indeed, if the view of Rowe and Kahn is valid, there is great promise that the functional loss found in many of the elderly can be circumvented.

REFERENCES

Bada, J. L., and Brown, S. E. (1980). Amino acid racemization in living mammals: Biochronological applications. *Trends Biochem. Sci,* 5, (9), iii–v.

Bates, S. R., and Gangloff, E. C. (1987). *Atherogenesis and Aging.* New York: Springer-Verlag.

Beaty, T. H., Cohen, B. H., Newill, C. A., Menken, H. A., Diamond, E. L., and Chen, C. J. (1982). Impaired pulmonary function as a risk factor for mortality. *Am. J. Epidemiol.,* 116, 102–13.

Belt, E. (1952). Leonardo da Vinci's studies of the aging process. *Geriatrics,* 7, 205–10.

Brandfonbrener, M., Landowne, M., and Shock, N. W. (1955). Changes in cardiac output with age. *Circulation,* 12, 557–66.

Brody, J. A., and Schneider, E. L. (1986). Diseases and disorders of aging: A hypothesis. *J. Chron. Dis.,* 39, 871–76.

Brown, W. T. (1985). Genetics of human aging. *Rev. Biol. Research in Aging,* 2, 105–16.

Burnet, F. M. (1970). An immunological approach into aging. *Lancet,* 2, 358–60.

Comfort, A. (1979). *The Biology of Senescence.* 3d ed. New York: Elsevier.

Costa, P. T., Jr., and McCrae, R. R. (1980). Functional age: A conceptual and empirical critique. In S. G. Haynes and M. Feinleib (Eds.), *Proc. Second Conf. Epidem. Aging.* NIH Publication 80–969.

Costa, P. T., Jr., and McCrae, R. R. (1985). Concepts of functional or biological age: A critical review. In R. Andres, E. L. Bierman, and W. R. Hazzard (Eds.), *Principles of Geriatric Medicine,* pp. 30–37. New York: McGraw-Hill.

Davies, D. F., and Shock, N. W. (1950). Age changes in glomerular filtration rate, effective renal plasma flow, and tubular excretory capacity in adult males. *J. Clin. Invest.* 29, 496–506.

Fries, J. F., and Crapo, L. M. (1981). *Vitality and Aging.* San Francisco: W. H. Freeman.

Garry, P. J., Goodwin, J. S., Hunt, W. C., Hooper, E. M., and Leonard, A. G. (1982). Nutritional status in a healthy elderly population: Dietary and supplemental intake. *Am. J. Clin. Nutr.,* 36, 319–31.

Goldman, R. (1977). Aging of the excretory system: Kidney and bladder. In C. E. Finch and L. Hayflick (Eds.), *Handbook of the Biology of Aging,* pp. 409–31. New York: Van Nostrand Reinhold.

Goodrick, C. (1975). Life-span and inheritance of longevity of inbred mice. *J. Geront.,* 30, 257–63.

Griffin, J. J. (1950). Aristotle's observations on gerontology. *Geriatrics,* 5, 222–26.

Harman, D. (1981). The aging process. *Proc. Natl. Acad. Sci. USA,* 78, 7124–28.

Hausman, P. B., and Weksler, M. E. (1985). Changes in the immune response with age. In C. E. Finch and E. L. Schneider (Eds.), *Handbook of the Biology of Aging.* 2d ed., pp. 414–32. New York: Van Nostrand Reinhold.

Hayflick, L., and Moorhead, P. S. (1961). The serial cultivation of human diploid cell strains. *Exp. Cell Res.,* 25, 585–621.

Kallman, E. J., and Jarvik, L. F. (1959). Individual differences in constitution and genetic background. In J. E. Birren (Ed.), *Handbook of Aging and the Individual,* p. 216. Chicago: University of Chicago Press.

Kannel, W. G. (1985). Hypertension and aging. In C. E. Finch and E. L. Schneider (Eds.), *Handbook of the Biology of Aging.* 2d ed., pp. 858–77. New York: Van Nostrand Reinhold.

Katzman, R. (1985). Aging and age-dependent diseases: Cognition and dementia. In *America's Aging: Health in an Older Society,* pp. 129–52. Washington, D.C.: National Academy Press.

Katzman, R., and Terry, R. (1983). Normal aging of the nervous system. In R. Katzman and R. Terry (Eds.), *Neurology of Aging,* pp. 15–49. Philadelphia: F. A. Davis.

Kirkwood, T.B.L. (1985). Comparative and evolutionary aspects of longevity. In C. E. Finch and E. L. Schneider (Eds.), *Handbook of the Biology of Aging.* 2d ed., pp. 27–44. New York: Van Nostrand Reinhold.

Kirkwood, T.B.L., and Holliday, R. (1979). The evaluation of aging and longevity. *Proc. Roy. Soc. Lond. Biol.,* 205, 531–46.

Kohn, R. R. (1978). *Principles of Mammalian Aging.* 2d ed. Englewood Cliffs, N.J.: Prentice-Hall.

Lakatta, E. G. (1985). Health, disease and cardiovascular aging. In *America's Aging: Health in an Older Society,* pp. 73–104. Washington, D.C.: National Academy Press.

Lang, C. A., and Richie, J. P., Jr. (1986). Biogerontological precepts of Nathan Shock which influenced our aging research. *Exper. Geront.,* 21, 235–39.

Lindeman, R. D., Tobin, J., and Shock, N. W. (1985). Longitudinal studies on the rate of decline in renal function with age. *J. Am. Geriatr. Soc.,* 33, 278–85.

Maeda, H., Gleiser, C. A., Masoro, E. J., Murata, I., McMahan, C. A., and Yu, B. P. (1985). Nutritional influences on aging of Fischer 344 rats: II. Pathology. *J. Geront.,* 40, 671–88.

Masoro, E. J. (1985). Nutrition and aging—A current assessment. *J. Nutr.,* 115, 842–48.

Masoro, E. J. (1986). Physiology of aging. In P. Holm-Pedersen and H. Löe (Eds.), *Geriatric Dentistry,* pp. 34–55. Copenhagen: Munksgaard.

Masoro, E. J. (1987a). Biology of aging: Current state of knowledge. *Arch. Intern. Med.,* 147, 166–69.

Masoro, E. J. (1987b). Criteria for aging/atherogenesis animal model. In S. V. Bates and E. C. Gangloff (Eds.), *Atherogenesis and Aging,* pp. 149–53. New York: Springer-Verlag.

Nohl, H., and Hegner, D. (1978). Do mitochondria produce oxygen radicals in vivo? *Eur. J. Biochem.,* 82, 563–67.

Norwood, T. H., and Smith, J. R. (1985). The cultured fibroblast-like cell as a model for the study of aging. In C. E. Finch and E. L. Schneider (Eds.), *Handbook of the Biology of Aging.* 2d ed., pp. 291–321. New York: Van Nostrand Reinhold.

Reff, M. E., and Schneider, E. L. (Eds.) (1982). *Biological Markers of Aging.* NIH Publication No. 82-2221.

Richardson, A., Roberts, M. S., and Rutherford, M. S. (1985). Aging and gene expression. *Rev. Biol. Res. in Aging,* 2, 395–419.

Rowe, J. W., and Kahn, R. L. (1987). Human aging: Usual and successful. *Science,* 237, 143–49.

Sacher, G. A. (1977). Life table modification and life prolongation. In C. E. Finch and L. Hayflick (Eds.), *Handbook of the Biology of Aging,* pp. 582–638. New York: Van Nostrand Reinhold.

Schneider, E. L., and Reed, J. D. (1985). Life extension. *N. Engl. J. Med.,* 312, 1159–68.

Schoenfeld, G. (1984). Atherosclerosis and plasma lipid transport with aging. In H. J. Armbrecht, J. M. Prendergast, and R. M. Coe (Eds.), *Nutritional Intervention in the Aging Process,* pp. 49–68. New York: Springer-Verlag.

Shock, N. W., and Yiengst, M. J. (1950). Age changes in the acid base equilibrium of the blood of males. *J. Geront.,* 5, 1–4.

Shock, N. W., and Yiengst, M. J. (1955). Age changes in respiratory measurements and metabolism in males. *J. Geront.* 10, 31–40.

Spirduso, W. W. (1974). Reaction and movement times as a function of age and physical activity level. *J. Geront.,* 30, 435–40.

Strehler, B. L. (1977). *Time, Cell, and Aging.* 2d ed. New York: Academic Press.

Strong, L. C. (1952). Observations on gerontology in the seventeenth century. *J. Geront.,* 7, 618–19.

Szilard, L. (1959). On the nature of the aging processes. *Proc. Natl. Sci. Acad. USA,* 45, 30–45.

Upton, A. C. (1977). Pathology. In C. E. Finch and L. Hayflick (Eds.), *Handbook of the Biology of Aging,* pp. 513–35. New York: Van Nostrand Reinhold.

3. THE PSYCHOLOGY OF ADULT DEVELOPMENT AND AGING: NEW APPROACHES AND METHODOLOGIES IN THE DEVELOPMENTAL STUDY OF COGNITION AND PERSONALITY

William J. Hoyer and Karen Hooker

The purpose of this chapter is to review selectively the recent work in several new research areas within the psychology of adult development and aging. We focus on new approaches and methodologies that seem particularly useful for the purpose of studying age-related changes in cognition, personality, health, and the interrelationships among these areas. In the cognitive area, we give special attention to: (1) intraindividual change and interindividual differences in the elementary perceptual and cognitive processes affecting the encoding, selection, and integration of information, and (2) intraindividual change and interindividual differences in knowledge availability, activation, and use. In the area of personality, we focus mainly on new developments in the study of intraindividual change and stability in personality during the adult life span. We also consider recent findings in the area of health behavior and aging, and new work bearing on the study of age-related changes in the interrelationships among personality, health, stress, and coping.

COGNITION AND AGING

Developmental change (and regularity) in cognition arises out of a reliance on accumulated knowledge or experience as well as from age-related changes in the elementary information processes and operations that control or limit the speed and efficiency of information acquisition, transformation, and use. Cognition does not show an orderly pattern of uni-dimensional change with advancing age. Within and across individuals, some mental abilities improve, some stay at roughly the same level, and some decline (e.g., see Baltes, 1987). Comprehensive theories in the area of cognitive aging must account for differential patterns of observable age-related gains and losses in various aspects of cognitive function. Given such diversity, we suggest the usefulness of models and methods that emphasize the analysis of *intraindividual change* and *interindividual differences* in intraindividual change. We begin this section by attempting to identify the major sources of age-related individual differences in cognitive function.

Level of cognitive performance (regardless of age) depends on a variety of factors including characteristics of the information being processed (e.g., its familiarity, salience, affective value, and complexity), the speed and efficiency of the elementary information processing skills required for performance, the ability to coordinate elementary processing operations, and the individual's ability to access and use task-relevant knowledge. As a way of organizing the burgeoning amount of literature on cognitive aging, we have grouped these factors into two broad classes as follows: (1) elementary and control processes involving the encoding, selection, and integration of information, and (2) processes that control availability, selection, and access to acquired knowledge. Below we review new directions in these research areas.

Elementary and Control Processes

It is generally assumed that the elementary operations of feature extraction, rate of information processing, memory search, and so on are involved in more complex cognitive processes and that the efficiency and speed of elementary operations should in part account for individual differences in complex cognitive performance. Cerella (1985) and Salthouse (1985) have been the primary advocates of the parsimonious view that most, if not all, age-related declines in cognitive tasks can be accounted for by a slowdown in the speed of execution of mental computations (but see Salthouse, in press).

The elementary processes of information extraction (Eriksen, Hamlin, and Breitmeyer, 1970), localization (Sekuler and Ball, 1986), processing rate (Cerella, 1985; Salthouse, 1985), perceptual search and selectivity (Madden, 1986; Plude and Hoyer, 1981, 1986), mental rotation and spatial integration (Berg, Hertzog, and Hunt, 1982; Cerella, Poon, and Fozard, 1981), speed of memory search and retrieval (Wickens, Braune, and Stokes, 1987), decision time under conditions of uncertainty (Hoyer and Familant, 1987; Rabbitt, 1982), and working memory (Charness, 1985; Hartley and Anderson, 1983; Light, Zelinski, and Moore, 1982; Reder, Wible, and Martin, 1986) all tend to be slower and/or less efficient in older adults as compared with younger adults. Further, the magnitude of age-related differences in elementary processing generally increases as load-type manipulations (i.e., increased task difficulty or complexity) are imposed. For example, most studies show that older adults are at a greater disadvantage compared with younger adults whenever limited processing resources have to be distributed among different tasks (e.g., Clancy and Hoyer, 1988; Craik, 1983; Madden, 1986; McDowd, 1986; Salthouse, in press). These findings suggest that older adults are at a disadvantage either when tasks compete for the same processing resources or when task efficiency depends on the ability to minimize competition between (or among) multiple processing demands. For example, Rabbitt (1982) suggested an age-related breakdown in the control processes associated with adjusting cognitive limitations to task demands. Craik (1983) provided a somewhat different explanation by suggesting that adult age differences in memory encoding and retrieval are a function of the extent to which self-initiated constructive operations are required. Craik pointed out that some encoding operations are so well practiced for some individuals on some tasks that the encoding is carried out largely automatically (i.e., without effort). Other encoding operations may require substantial self-initiated effort, in which case age reductions in memory performance would be apparent. Retrieval tasks can also vary in the degree to which they require effort and self-initiated constructive processes. For example, free recall tasks provide minimal environmental or contextual support and a high degree of self-initiated activity, whereas certain types of recognition and priming tasks are highly context-supported and require relatively little self-generated cognitive activity.

Studies of semantic priming and aging, in which words are used to "automatically" activate a network of related words and meanings, typically show negligible age differences (Chiarello, Church, and Hoyer, 1985; Howard, McAndrews, and Lasaga, 1981). Note, however, that there can be individual differences in the retrieval processes associated with using contextual information to facilitate knowledge access (e.g., Moscovitch, Winocur, and McLachlan, 1986) and in the extent to which certain information is accessible or available through priming (e.g, Clancy and Hoyer, 1988). In contrast to Craik's position that adult age differences in memory reflect different degrees of self-initiated constructive operations, Light and Singh (1987) and others (e.g., Howard, in press; Chiarello and Hoyer, in press) have suggested that age differences in memory may involve the operation of different (or disassociated) memory systems (e.g., see also Sherry and Schacter, 1987).

Independent of the issue of disassociability of memory systems, most researchers agree that the control process function is a prime locus of aging differences on tasks that require the integration of new information, active memory search, and/or the coordination of other capacity-demanding processes. Although older adults are generally not at a disadvantage with regard to the execution of highly practiced skills, the sequencing and coordination of such skills are frequently affected by age. Intraindividual change or variability across measurement occasions in cognitive performance may be largely a function of fluctuations in the operations of control processes (e.g., see Salthouse, Kausler, and Saults, 1986).

Knowledge Accessibility and Use

Based in part on recent notions of the modularity of cognitive organization (e.g., Fodor, 1983; Marshall, 1984), it has been suggested that age-related gains and losses in different types or dimensions of cognition can be explained in terms of reduced plasticity and increased domain-specificity of knowledge access (Hoyer, 1987; Hoyer, Rybash, and Roodin, 1988; Rybash, Hoyer, and Roodin, 1986). In contrast to the well-established age-related reductions in the efficiency of elementary and control processes, cognitive proficiency in the later years can be maintained or even enhanced in "skilled domains." Such maintenance or enhancement can be attributed to the efficiency of domain-specific encoding or retrieval processes and/or to the amount of contextual support (e.g., priming, cuing) available in well-practiced cognitive tasks. Also, Glaser (1984) has pointed out that it is frequently more important to be able to retrieve knowledge appropriate to the task demands than to be able to rapidly execute mental computations in everyday cognitive tasks. Rybash, Hoyer, and Roodin (1986) suggested that cognitive performance in adulthood depends in part on the possession and judicious use of acquired knowledge, and on the ability to make inferences and deductions based on extant knowledge schemes.

Some writers have suggested that cognitive growth during childhood and early adulthood is associated with increased speed of mental computations, enlarged mental capacity, and improved access to knowledge (e.g., see Chi, 1985; Kail and Bisanz, 1982; Perlmutter, in press; Sternberg, in press). By extension, this view has implications for the understanding of cognitive development during the later adult years. On the one hand, knowledge and understanding develop cumulatively; and, on the other hand, there are declines in the general speed and efficiency of computational operations which affect information encoding, transformation, and retrieval with aging. However, it may be useful to distinguish between the acquisition of *new* computational processes and the execution or use of well-learned computational processes; the former show substantial age-related decline compared to the latter which are relatively age-invariant. Hoyer, Rybash, and Roodin (1988) suggested that adult cognitive development is characterized by growth of and ease of access to domain-specific knowledge. Although acquisition of knowledge is basic to cognitive development throughout the life span, it seems that strategies of knowledge access become more robust and applicable to a wider range of tasks during childhood and up through the early adulthood years. However, acquired strategies of knowledge access may become largely task-bound and content-specific during the later adult years.

Recently, Charness (in press) has reviewed the work on cognitive expertise and age. The general finding is that older adults continue to function as experts in mastered domains despite apparent losses in some of the component information-processing abilities. Salthouse (1984), for example, reported that typing speed was uncorrelated with age for skilled typists, despite the expected negative correlations between age and standard psychomotor reaction time performance. Salthouse suggested that older skilled typists compensate for age-related declines in speed and reaction time on the typing task by looking farther ahead within the window of available text, thereby giving more time to plan the execution of keystrokes. Salthouse's findings illustrate the domain-specific nature of skilled performance, since skilled typists did not employ the "look ahead" strategy on the digit symbol substitution test or other tasks.

With aging, individuals are able to maintain or extend the range and depth of cognitive expertise in some domains more so than in others. For example, performance in physically demanding types of work or sport eventually declines with age even for those who manifest expert performance in young adulthood (e.g., Backman and Molander, 1986). But performance in cognitive domains that allow more time for planning, knowledge utilization, and retrieval may continue to improve with age and experience well into the seventh or eighth decades of life.

Related to the notion of domains of knowledge is the concept of "scripts." Scripts are representations of learned information, such as how to solve arithmetic problems or how to order food in a restaurant. Scripts begin as generalized memory structures, which then become elaborated and transformed into generalized event representations. The construction and elaboration of scripts is considered to be a control process, the efficiency of which varies with age and other ability-related individual difference factors. The efficiency of execution of well-learned scripts is unaffected by age-related decrements in elementary processes or in various control functions such as information integration. There is empirical evidence to support the distinction between the acquisition and the execution of scripted material. For example, the task of actually computing the product of twelve times twenty is different than the act of "automatically" producing the memorized solution to twelve times twelve (Jacoby, 1978). Age differences are found mainly in the computational processes and not in execution of well-learned knowledge (see Charness, in press; Hasher and Zacks, 1979; Hoyer, 1987).

New Theoretical Developments

Thus far, we have briefly described age-related changes in some of the processes involved in acquiring and using knowledge. It is clear that there are reliable age-related declines in several important aspects of information processing, learning, and memory. Although researchers are seldom able to pinpoint the specific mechanisms responsible for cognitive decline, the research has illuminated the kinds of abilities and processes that are most age-sensitive. Further, a relatively clear picture has emerged in recent years with regard to the conditions under which age-related declines are most likely to be found. General decline and differential decline (indicated by interactions involving age with task complexity, information load, and/or effort) are usually explained in terms of age-related limitations in mental capacity, mental resources, or speed of processing. Salthouse (1988, in press) has argued that the invocation of such accounts actually explains very little, if anything, about the nature of age-related decline. As researchers become more precise in their operationalization of such concepts as capacity and resources, and as they begin to develop and use task-independent measures of cognitive capacity, circularity in theory-building will become less of a problem for the field.

Many of the available explanations of cognitive growth during the adult years are also unsatisfactory (e.g., Baltes, 1987). The thrust of much of the work emphasizing the positive aspects of cognitive functioning in the later years has been to discount the studies showing age declines in information processing and intelligence on the basis that there is age bias in the measures used. Age differences in the effects of demand characteristics on cognitive performance should be taken into account in evaluating the size of the age difference between young and old. However, it is also important to consider the possibility that different types of intelligence may characterize different developmental periods. That is, many of the unique attributes of adult cognitive competence are not captured by the available models and measures of adult cognition, since older adults are compared to young on measures designed to assess the attributes of intelligence and cognition that young people are likely to possess. Unlike the tasks typically studied in the psychology laboratory, many of the cognitive tasks of everyday life are open-ended, and knowledge or experience is frequently applied in a nonlogical, relativistic, and/or dialectic manner. Recently, several writers have extended or modified aspects of standard Piagetian theory so as to capture some of the unique and salient characteristics of adult forms of thought (e.g., Arlin, 1984; Basseches, 1984; Koplowitz, 1984; Labouvie-Vief, 1984). This work has been particularly useful for the purposes of: (1) calling attention to positive dimensions of cognitive development, (2) emphasizing nonlogical aspects of cognition, and (3) describing features (or products) of some of the unique forms of adult cognition such as problem-finding, relativistic thinking, creativity, and dialectical thinking.

Arlin (1984), for example, described the problem-finding mode, which she contrasted with the problem-solving quality of formal thought. Koplowitz (1984) argued that postformal thinking embraced the principles of nonlinear causality, the complete interdependence (and nonseparability) of variables, the open nature of boundaries and systems, and the existence of self-constructed entities and objects within a self-constructed and contextual world. In contrast, he noted that Piaget's model of formal thinking embraced the principles of linear causality, independence and separation of variables, the closed nature of systems and boundaries, and the existence of permanent/stable entities and objects within a stable external world. Basseches (1984) has emphasized the dialectical qualities of postformal thought, such as the ability to: (1) accept contradiction as a basic facet of physical and social reality, (2) appreciate the holistic and constitutive nature of one's knowledge systems, and (3) conceptualize reality, as well as knowledge of reality, within an open and self-evolving framework. Indeed, these are some of the positive characteristics of adult cognition.

There have been some new and useful developments related to the conceptualization of cognitive aging. Some of these conceptual advances have been brought about by new methodologies and procedures for the analysis of age-related change, and some appear as recastings or revisions of long-standing research problems in the study of adult development and aging. In 1958, for example, Welford reported that one of the most reliable findings in the cognitive aging research literature was that there is increased interindividual variability as we move along the adult age continuum. Many recent studies continue to call attention to the "problem" of age-related increases in interindividual and intraindividual variability in various aspects of cognitive functioning (e.g., Hertzog, 1985; Hoyer, 1974; Karuza and Zevon, 1985; Salthouse, Kausler, and Saults, 1986). Based on the research we have reviewed here, it seems reasonable to suggest that diverse or unique intraindividual patterns of age-related gains and losses in different aspects of cognition can be described in terms of a narrowing of the range of effective cognitive function and a continued strengthening (or maintenance) of cognitive functioning within selected cognitive domains. Environmental influences as well as neurobiological antecedents affect individual performance, which suggests the use of *P*-technique and other analytic approaches suitable for the study of patterns of change based on multiple measures recorded over many occasions of observation. We discuss this approach in detail later in this chapter.

Toward an Integrative Approach

In recent years, new methods and approaches have been brought to bear on the fundamental issues of (1) defining the appropriate dimensions or markers of age and cohort (e.g., Featherman and Lerner, 1985; Schaie, 1986); (2) distinguishing the effects of age and health on behavior (Rodin, 1986; Rowe and Kahn, 1987); and (3) representing the role of experience, skill, or "wisdom" in aging (e.g., Baltes, 1987). A paradox becomes apparent when such issues are examined. That is, one of the puzzling aspects in studying cognitive change in the later years is that growth or gains are frequently evident against a background of age-normative losses in basic cognitive function—at least as measured by standard intelligence tests or laboratory tasks. Rabbitt (1977) posed the problem as follows: "In view of the deterioration of memory and perceptual motor performance with advancing age, the right kind of question may well be not 'why are old people so bad at cognitive tasks' but rather 'how, in spite of growing disabilities, do old people preserve such relatively good performance?' " (p. 623). The task of cognitive aging researchers is further confused by the fact that abilities are simultaneously outcomes of past experience or learning (i.e., cognitive gains) and determinants of new learning (i.e., information processing abilities). That mental abilities are both antecedents and outcomes of the developing individual's experience suggests the usefulness of taking an integrative approach to the study of adult cognitive development and aging. One such approach to model-building involves an integration of the two factors that we have discussed in this chapter. These are: (1) age-related declines in the ability to initiate the processes that encode, organize, compute, and transform information (e.g., Craik, 1983); (2) either age-invariance or gain in the availability, accessibility, or use of domain-specific knowledge.

PERSONALITY AND AGING

Since there are recent comprehensive reviews of research and theory in the area of adult personality development (e.g., Bengtson, Reedy, and Gordon, 1985; McCrae and Costa, 1984), our aim in this section is to discuss newly emerging research areas that we think will prove to be particularly fruitful for understanding the development of personality in adulthood. We also discuss several conceptual and methodological issues that bear on the study of these newly emerging research areas.

One important research issue involves the extent to which there is change in personality during the adult life span. Interest in this question probably stems from the desire to predict what people of a given age will be like in subsequent years. Is one likely to remain the same as one is at present? If there are changes, are they patterned in such a way as to be predictable? If change is possible, but not certain, what life experiences are likely to trigger change? These are important questions because the answers imply different strategies for individuals to use in developing plans, goals, and coping functions.

Ordered Change versus Stability

The most comprehensive theories of personality development in adulthood are those that emphasize *ordered changes* in self and personality throughout life (e.g., Buhler, 1968; Erikson, 1950; Gould, 1978; Jung, 1933; Levinson et al., 1978; Loevinger, 1976; Vaillant, 1977). However, there is little evidence to support theories of universal stages of adult personality development (Datan, Rodeheaver, and Hughes, 1987). Instead, changes are often multidirectional and specific to certain groups of individuals—features antithetical to the emphases of stage theories on linearity, universality, irreversibility, and end-state orientation (Baltes and Nesselroade, 1979). Although adulthood is age-graded to some extent (Hagestad and Neugarten, 1985), development encompasses many role changes (e.g., marriage), nonnormative life events (e.g., living in another culture), and contexts for development (e.g., work environments) that are *not* tied to the number of years since birth (e.g., see Schaie, 1986). Thus, chronologic age may not be the best variable to use for describing intraindividual personality development. For example, phase of the family life cycle may be a more potent predictor of personality for women than age per se (e.g., Reinke, Ellicott, Harris, and Hancock, 1985).

Another major framework for the study of personality in adulthood is trait theory, as exemplified in the work of Costa and McCrae (1980a). Trait theorists view personality as an enduring and relatively stable set of dispositions (e.g.,

Livson, 1973). Traits are derived from factor analyses of responses to items designed to sample the entire realm of personality.

Costa and McCrae (e.g., 1978; Costa, McCrae, and Arenberg, 1980) have conducted an impressive array of studies that support the notion that there are stable individual differences in the trait clusters of *neuroticism, extraversion,* and *openness to experience*. McCrae and Costa (1987) have recently added the dimensions of *agreeableness* and *conscientiousness* to their model, and they have developed the NEO Personality Inventory as the instrument to measure this five-factor model of personality (Costa and McCrae, 1985).

While recognizing the contribution of the trait framework, it is important to point out that the trait approach does not specify how stable individual differences develop or how early in life they stabilize. Descriptions of whether or not traits change yield limited information. More important for understanding personality processes and development is determining the extent of plasticity of personality and identifying the *mechanisms* that promote change or maintain stability. It is just as important to determine *why* stability is exhibited when change might reasonably be expected as it is to determine why change occurs. According to Nesselroade and Ford (1985), manifestations of individual differences are like "fossils" in that they signify the operation of different processes or that different outcomes have been produced by the same process, but they themselves give no indication of the nature of these processes.

Types of Stability and Aging

Claims for stability or change with age must be evaluated with respect to *which type* of stability has been examined. Following Mortimer, Finch, and Kumka (1982), temporal stability can be conceived of in terms of: (1) structural invariance, (2) normative stability, (3) level stability, and (4) ipstative stability. Each of these represents a unique aspect of stability. *Structural invariance* refers to lack of structural or qualitative changes in dimensions studied. It is essential to establish equivalence of constructs (and measures) over time before attempting to make quantitative comparisons of the constructs at different ages (Nesselroade, 1977). Thus, demonstrating structural invariance is a prerequisite for examining other types of stability. *Normative stability* refers to the retention of individual ranking on a certain characteristic over time, relative to some reference group. Studies that report correlation coefficients between the same construct at different ages are informative with respect to normative stability. Many studies of personality in adulthood have shown correlation coefficients that are quite high over a period of many years (e.g., Block, 1971; Britton and Britton, 1972; Conley, 1985; Costa and McCrae, 1978; Costa, McCrae, and Arenberg, 1980; Finn, 1986; Kelly, 1955; Leon, Gillum, Gillum, and Gouze, 1979; Siegler, George, and Okun, 1979; Skolnick, 1966; Tuddenham, 1959). However, researchers should not make the mistake of arguing that the data show that people did not change, since this type of assessment does not address absolute level. For example, if most people become more introspective with age (Neugarten, 1968) but many retain their relative ranking on this variable with respect to the sample as a whole, normative stability would be demonstrated although everyone in the sample may have shown intraindividual change. *Level stability* refers to invariance of mean level over time. The relatively few studies of the absolute level of stability of adult personality have yielded a pattern of mixed results. Block (1971), Britton and Britton (1972), Haan, Millsap, and Hartka (1986), Kelly (1955), Leon et al. (1979), and Stevens and Truss (1985) reported significant changes in mean level of personality attributes. Costa and McCrae (1978), Schaie and Parham (1976), and Siegler et al. (1979) found little evidence of change in mean level. *Ipstative stability* refers to intraindividual change over time. It is ironic that researchers have paid least attention to this type of stability given that the primary goal of developmental research is to study interindividual differences in intraindividual change (Baltes, Reese, and Nesselroade, 1977). When ipsative stability has been studied (e.g., Block, 1971; Britton and Britton, 1972; Maas and Kuypers, 1975), it has been shown that some individuals were extremely stable while others exhibited a great deal of personality change.

Methodological Issues

Conflicting findings regarding age-related interindividual differences in the patterns of change and stability in adult personality call attention to several important methodological issues in the study of developmental change. Theorists who argue for ordered change are more likely to rely on qualitative methods such as open-ended interviews and projective tests. Perhaps such methods are ones most conducive to illuminating changes. Methodological flaws associated with these types of measures include interviewer bias and limited information on validity and reliability (see McCrae and Costa, 1984, for a critique).

Alternatively, trait theorists who use questionnaire instruments to gather data may be underestimating change. In the development of psychometrically sound, standardized tests, items that do not correlate highly over time (i.e., do not show high test-retest reliability) are usually eliminated. However, when studying change it is important to separate measurement reliability from lability of the construct being measured. The test-retest correlation coefficient confounds these two sources of variance. It is possible to reliably measure a labile construct (see Nesselroade, Pruchno, and Jacobs, 1986).

Also problematic from the standpoint of evaluating change is that some instruments include questions about the individual's past, which obviously cannot change if respondents are truthful at all testing occasions (McClelland, 1980). For example, an item on the Psychopathy Scale of the MMPI is, "During one period when I was a youngster I engaged in petty thievery." A person who responds "true" to such a statement must make this same response no matter how many times the test is administered—even though the respondent may *now* be an exemplary citizen. Therefore, this item will show high reliability but a lack of sensitivity to changes in people. Thus, theorists working within a trait framework using standardized questionnaires may be most likely to find that personality is stable.

The hypothesis that researchers using qualitative methods may be more likely to discover changes in personality while researchers using instruments designed to measure traits may be more likely to find stability in personality is a speculative "explanation" of mixed findings, perhaps worthy of empirical research through a technique such as meta-analysis (Rosenthal, 1984). In any such undertaking one should attend to the numerous methodological issues, such as selective attrition, time between measurements, examination of cohort and time of measurement effects, population studied, and so on (e.g., see McCrae and Costa, 1984, for a summary of these issues).

Measurement of Intraindividual Change

A new methodological approach in the study of personality in adulthood involves the use of multivariate, replicated, single-subject designs that focus on intraindividual change (e.g., Hooker, 1985; Nesselroade, 1988; Nesselroade and Ford, 1985). Although life span developmentalists purport to seek understanding of intraindividual change and interindividual differences and similarities in intraindividual change (e.g., Baltes, Reese, and Nesselroade, 1977), there has been relatively little research on intraindividual change processes (Hoyer, 1974). Labouvie (1982) pointed out that most research is focused on the study of changes in interindividual differences (group approach) rather than the person-centered approach of differences in intraindividual changes. "By relating interindividual differences at any one point in time to differences at other points in time via means-averages or correlations-covariances, it is change in interindividual differences rather than differences in intraindividual change that is constructed and interpreted" (Labouvie, 1982, p. 60).

There are several reasons why intraindividual change is an important domain for research: (1) Recognition of the increasing heterogeneity found in older populations (e.g., Rowe and Kahn, 1987) calls for research that traces individual developmental trajectories to discover how individuals become so different from one another. (2) Gerontologists have long recognized the importance of studying person-context relationships (e.g., Lawton and Nahemow, 1973) which necessarily take place at the *individual,* not group, level (Epstein, 1983; Pervin, 1983). Both person characteristics and aspects of the context hypothesized to be related to the person must be sampled over multiple occasions. (3) A focus on the individual, also known as the idiographic approach, is regaining respect among personality researchers (e.g., Bem and Allen, 1974; Kenrick and Dantchik, 1983; Pervin, 1983; Runyan, 1983). This approach seems especially appropriate for the study of older adults, given the heterogeneity of this population (Rowe and Kahn, 1987). (4) Recently, it has been argued that individuals actively construct and continuously reconstruct their personalities throughout the life course (e.g.,

Cohler, 1982; Datan, Rodeheaver, and Hughes, 1987; Ryff, 1984; Whitbourne, 1985). From this perspective, individuals are continually "rewriting" their past to make their life a coherent story. According to Datan et al. (1987) a life story is "an attempt by the individual to create a narrative, given order and predictability only by the choices and decision-making of that individual. The order in the course of lives lies, then, in the minds of the persons experiencing those lives, not in the observer" (pp. 162–63). The study of life stories obviously requires an idiographic approach since it would not make sense to "average" stories together to yield a general life story. Researchers can rely on archival material, such as letters, in addition to the subject's own narrative. Although such data are qualitative, quantitative procedures are available to aid interpretation.

As mentioned earlier, one quantitative approach for the study of intraindividual change along multiple measures is P-technique (e.g., see Nesselroade and Ford, 1985). P-technique involves obtaining measures on many occasions (preferably one hundred or more) for multiple variables for one individual. The measurements obtained on the variables are intercorrelated over occasions and then factored in the usual manner. The factors represent dimensions of differences within the individual, i.e., intraindividual change. Information on the relationship of the change dimensions to time can then be examined using a multivariate time-series analytic strategy (e.g., Molenaar, 1985).

P-technique studies focus on the examination of intraindividual change (e.g., Hooker, Nesselroade, Nesselroade, and Lerner, 1987; Lebo and Nesselroade, 1978; Zevon and Tellegen, 1982). By conducting several concurrent replications of the study (i.e., collecting P-technique data for multiple subjects), one can examine interindividual differences and similarities in intraindividual change. Thus, the data are examined in a way that preserves the organization of personality within the individual and yet can address the issue of commonality in intraindividual change patterns by examining several subjects. A recent study by Hooker (1985) may be particularly interesting to gerontologists because she examined older adults going through the transition to retirement. There was evidence for intraindividual change factors in both personality and perceived context, and these domains were related to each other.

Personality and Health

It is important to consider the interrelationships among health, personality, and age in order to distinguish changes attributable to "normal aging" from changes associated with disease processes. The differential distribution of health over the life span poses challenging methodological problems in sampling from populations of different ages (Siegler, Nowlin, and Blumenthal, 1980). Most older adults have at least one chronic health problem (Soldo, 1980), whereas chronic health problems are relatively rare among younger adults. Health is the major predictor of well-being in later life (e.g., Larson, 1978) and, obviously, has pervasive effects on behavior. Therefore, it is important to understand the relationship between health and personality and how relationships between these domains may change over the life span.

Although there are many studies on the relationship between disease and personality (e.g., Booth-Kewley and Friedman, 1987; Friedman and Booth-Kewley, 1987), there are only a few studies on how the relationships between personality and health are related to aging. For example, Costa and McCrae (1980b) found that adults high in neuroticism tend to complain more about their health and are more likely to smoke and have drinking problems than those adults low in neuroticism. Smoking and excessive drinking are related to disease (e.g., cancer, heart disease), suggesting an indirect link between the personality dimension of neuroticism and poor health.

One area in which the relationship between personality and health has been studied extensively is that of the Type A behavior pattern (TABP) and coronary heart disease (CHD). The Type A construct was first described by cardiologists Friedman and Rosenman (1959), who were convinced that early onset of CHD was linked to a style of behavior. Components of the TABP include excessive competitive striving, time urgency, aggressiveness, and hostility. Friedman and Rosenman (1974) described the Type A person as one who "is aggressively involved in a chronic, incessant struggle to achieve more and more in less and less time, and if required to do so, against the opposing efforts of other things or other persons" (p. 67). A person who lacks the exaggerated Type A characteristics is known as Type B.

Prospective data from the Western Collaborative Group Study (Rosenman et al., 1975) and the Framingham Heart Study (Haynes, Feinleib, and Kannel, 1980) led a panel of experts to conclude that employed, middle-aged U.S. citizens who display the TABP are more likely to develop CHD than their Type B counterparts. However, there are recent studies showing no relationship between CHD and TABP (e.g., Case, Heller, Case, and Moss, 1985; Shekelle, Gale, and Norusis, 1985). Such inconsistencies across studies underscore the importance of determining *which aspect(s)* of the TABP are predictive of CHD, in which *populations* using which *measures* of TABP (Matthews and Haynes, 1986). For example, there is emerging consensus that hostility and anger are the "toxic" components of TABP—i.e., those most predictive of CHD (Barefoot, Dahlstrom, and Williams, 1983; Dembroski, MacDougall, Williams, Haney, and Blumenthal, 1985; Williams et al., 1980).

Williams et al. (1986) offered both new evidence to support the link between TABP and angiographically documented coronary atherosclerosis and an intriguing explanation for the inconsistent findings reported in the literature. They postulated that the TABP decreases in importance as a risk factor with increasing age. Thus, samples that include older subjects may obscure the relationship between TABP and disease found among younger subjects. Williams et al. (1986) pointed out that the angiographic studies reporting negative results all included patients ranging up to sixty-four to seventy years of age. Their results on a large sample of coronary angiography patients suggested an interaction between age and Type A/B. Type A patients aged forty-five or younger had more severe atherosclerosis than did Type B patients; whereas among older patients (age fifty-five and older), there was a slight trend toward more severe disease among Type Bs. Williams et al. (1986) noted that selective attrition may account for these findings. That is, as the biologically vulnerable Type As become deceased, longitudinal samples become increasingly overrepresented by "hardy" Type As.

Longitudinal data extending from middle age to later life are necessary to test the biological hardiness hypothesis. However, cross-sectional data indicate that this is a reasonable hypothesis, since there are disproportionately few older adults who can be categorized as strong Type As (Howard, Rechnitzer, Cunningham, and Donner, 1986; Siegler et al., 1987). There is some support for the "hardiness" hypothesis from a recent longitudinal study by Barefoot et al. (1987). They found that scores on Factor L of the 16 PF, a measure of suspiciousness closely related to hostility measures, predicted mortality among participants of the Duke Second Longitudinal Study. It should be noted, however, that although suspiciousness predicted mortality, it did not predict death from CHD more strongly than death from other causes. In fact, these results are consistent with conclusions drawn from a meta-analysis by Friedman and Booth-Kewley (1987). These authors found support for the notion of a *generic* "disease prone personality" and found relatively little evidence suggesting that *specific* personality factors (e.g., hostility) lead to *specific* disease end states (e.g., CHD).

Another way of examining relationships between personality and health is to view personality as a resistance resource that can buffer the individual from the negative health consequences of stress (Kobasa, Maddi, and Kahn, 1982). Kobasa et al. (1982) argued that personality dispositions bias one toward experiencing stimuli in a particular way (e.g., personality affects cognitive appraisal) and also serve to energize a particular set of coping activities. Kobasa and her colleagues (Kobasa, 1979; Kobasa et al., 1982; Kobasa, Maddi, and Zola, 1983; Kobasa and Puccetti, 1983) have advanced the notion of a hardy personality, which consists of high levels of commitment, challenge, and perceived control. Kobasa et al. (1982) prospectively demonstrated that hardy individuals have fewer illness symptoms than individuals low in hardiness. Kobasa et al. (1982) suggested that commitment, challenge, and control affect health by being associated with decreased use of ineffective coping strategies.

Recent studies show that hardiness may not be a unitary phenomenon (Hull, Van Treuren, and Virnelli, 1987) and that the subcomponents of commitment and control are directly responsible for the association of hardiness with health outcomes (e.g., Funk and Houston, 1987). Whether personality influences coping strategies for reducing stress (indirect link) or whether certain personality characteristics are stressful per se (direct link), it seems clear that personality and health are related via stress.

Stress and Coping

Antonovsky (1979), Coelho, Hamburg, and Adams (1974), and Lazarus and Folkman (1984) provided excellent reviews of the literature on stress and coping.

Stress occurs when the demands of situation are perceived to exceed one's resources for coping. Stress can result from major life events (Holmes and Rahe, 1967), the ordinary hassles of everyday living (DeLongis, Coyne, Dakof, Folkman, and Lazarus, 1982), and chronic life strains (Pearlin, Lieberman, Menaghan, and Mullan, 1981). However, it is how people cope with stress, rather than stress per se that affects health (e.g., Billings and Moos, 1981; Pearlin and Schooler, 1978).

According to Folkman and Lazarus (1980), "Coping is defined as the cognitive and behavioral efforts made to master, tolerate, or reduce external and internal demands and conflicts among them" (p. 223). Some research has been directed at the question of whether older adults use different coping strategies than young adults. Studies show that older adults tend to use more passive, emotion-focused coping strategies (e.g., Felton and Revenson, 1987; Folkman, Lazarus, Pimley, and Novacek, 1987; Pearlin and Schooler, 1978; Quayhagen and Quayhagen, 1982) while younger adults tend to use more active, problem-focused coping strategies. However, Folkman and Lazarus (1980) and McCrae (1982) found that age differences in coping could be attributed to the nature of the stressor rather than age. The elderly tend to experience fewer, but more negative and uncontrollable, stressors (Folkman and Lazarus, 1980), which makes it more likely that coping would be emotion-focused rather than problem-focused.

Lazarus and DeLongis (1983) argued eloquently for the necessity of the intraindividual longitudinal research strategy in studying coping, especially among the elderly. *P*-technique would seem to be an ideal research strategy for this approach to the study of stress and coping. For example, one could target an upcoming stressful event (e.g., undergoing major surgery) and measure coping style and aspects of the context over multiple occasions. *P*-technique would allow one to examine intraindividual changes in coping strategies as they relate to contextual changes. For example, if one could show that a positive coping strategy such as information seeking increased on days that the patient had visitors, this could be useful information for medical staff.

Studies of stress and coping, with particular emphases on stressors of importance to the elderly, such as chronic illness (e.g., Felton and Revenson, 1987) and financial strain (e.g., Krause, 1987), are appearing in the literature. These studies, as well as studies of psychological hardiness and the Type A behavior pattern, are adding to our knowledge of the relationship between personality and health.

Personal Control and Health

Recent research is improving our understanding of the complex relationship between control and health. Generally, lack of control has been associated with poor mental and physical health outcomes (e.g., Rodin, 1986; Seligman, 1975). Rodin (1986) has argued that the relationship between control and health becomes stronger with increasing age, and she presented three rationales for the strength of this relationship in later life. First, control is more likely to be an issue in old age. Losses associated with aging, such as loss of spouse, friends, or retirement, effect what outcomes can be attained. These losses can also deprive the elderly of social interactions in which they get feedback regarding their competence. Second, indicators of health status are related to age. For example, there is a general loss of immunologic competence among the elderly. To the extent that processes related to control affect immunologic functioning, one may see an increase in the relationship of health and control with age. Finally, the extent to which a person has contact with the health care system may affect control, since the medical care system is one in which personal control is usually restricted. The more frequent contact of elderly persons with the medical system may exacerbate the effects of these restrictions on feelings of control.

It has been shown that interventions designed to increase control have positive effects on health (e.g., Langer and Rodin, 1976; Schulz, 1976). However, as Rodin (1986) pointed out, most of these studies have been in nursing homes, and there is little knowledge of the relationship between control and health among healthy, community-dwelling older adults. Also, it appears that loss of control has more negative effects than initial lack of control (e.g., Schulz and Hanusa, 1978), so interventions to enhance control must be maintained over time.

Rodin (1986) presented evidence from many studies that indicates that control directly affects health by changing the individual's pathophysiological processes, such as the level of circulating catecholamines and immune system functioning. She also argued that people high in perceived control may be more likely to engage in positive health behaviors that would result in better health. The study of health behavior among older adults is a new area of study (e.g., Siegler and Costa, 1985) and one that deserves increasing attention among gerontologic researchers.

CONCLUSION

The goal of this chapter is to briefly present the current thinking on issues of cognition and personality in later adulthood. Since health is a ubiquitous concern in later life, it is important to understand relationships between health and cognitive functioning as well as health and personality. Although relationships between health and cognitive functioning have been studied for some time (e.g., Spieth, 1965), new developments in psychophysiological instrumentation permit more careful analysis of these relationships. Although the study of health and personality in later life has a relatively shorter history, this area of research has also benefited from recent technological and methodological advances. Studies of the relationships among all three domains (health, personality, and cognition) are needed, but these require substantial scientific expertise and the resources of interdisciplinary collaboration.

A major theme of this chapter is that theoretical advancement in terms of understanding the heterogeneity of the elderly population will require an emphasis on new methodological approaches. Specifically, we suggested that research strategies that focus on intraindividual change will be useful for the purposes of explaining the multidimensional nature of cognitive and personality change in later life.

REFERENCES

Antonovsky, A. (1979). *Health, Stress, and Coping*. San Francisco: Jossey-Bass.

Arlin, P. K. (1984). Adolescent and adult thought: A structural interpretation. In M. L. Commons, F. A. Richards, and C. Armon (Eds.), *Beyond Formal Operations: Late Adolescent and Adult Cognitive Development*, pp. 258–71. New York: Praeger.

Backman, L., and Molander, B. (1986). Effects of adult age and level of skill on the ability to cope with high-stress conditions in a precision sport. *Psychology and Aging*, 1, 334–36.

Baltes, P. B. (1987). Theoretical propositions of life-span developmental psychology: On the dynamics between growth and decline. *Developmental Psychology*, 23, 611–26.

Baltes, P. B., and Lindenberger, U. (1988). On the range of cognitive plasticity in old age as a function of experience: Fifteen years of intervention research. *Behavior Therapy*, 19 (3), pp, 283–300.

Baltes, P. B., and Nesselroade, J. R. (1979). History and rationale of longitudinal research. In J. R. Nesselroade and P. B. Baltes (Eds.), *Longitudinal Research in the Study of Behavior and Development*, pp. 1–39. New York: Academic Press.

Baltes, P. B., Reese, H. W., and Nesselroade, J. R. (1977). *Life-Span Developmental Psychology: Introduction to Research Methods*. Monterey, Calif.: Brooks/Cole.

Barefoot, J. C., Dahlstrom, W. G., and Williams, R. B. (1983). Hostility, CHD incidence and total mortality: A 25-year follow-up study of 255 physicians. *Psychosomatic Medicine*, 45, 59–63.

Barefoot, J. C., Siegler, I. C., Nowlin, J. B., Peterson, B. L., Haney, T. L., and Williams, R. B. (1987). Suspiciousness, health, and mortality: A follow-up study of 500 older adults. *Psychosomatic Medicine*, 49, 450–57.

Basseches, M. (1984). Dialectical thinking as a metasystematic form of cognitive organization. In M. L. Commons, F. A. Richards, and C. Armon (Eds.), *Beyond Formal Operations: Late Adolescent and Adult Cognitive Development*, pp. 216–38. New York: Praeger.

Bem, D. J., and Allen, A. (1974). On predicting some of the people some of the time: The search for cross-situational consistencies in behavior. *Psychological Review*, 81, 506–20.

Bengtson, V. L., Reedy, M. N., and Gordon, C. (1985). Aging and self-conceptions: Personality processes and social contexts. In J. E. Birren and K. W. Schaie (Eds.), *Handbook of the Psychology of Aging*. 2d ed., pp. 544–93. New York: Van Nostrand Reinhold.

Berg, C., Hertzog, C. K., and Hunt, E. (1982). Age differences in the speed of mental rotation. *Developmental Psychology*, 18, 95–107.

Billings, A. G., and Moos, R. H. (1981). The role of coping responses and social resources in attenuating the impact of stressful life events. *Journal of Behavioral Medicine*, 4, 139–57.

Block, J. (1971). *Lives through Time*. Berkeley, Calif.: Bancroft Books.

Booth-Kewley, S., and Friedman, H. S. (1987). Psychological predictors of heart disease: A quantitative review. *Psychological Bulletin,* 101, 343–62.

Britton, J. H., and Britton, J. O. (1972). *Personality Changes in Aging: A Longitudinal Study of Community Residents.* New York: Springer.

Buhler, C. (1968). The developmental structure of goal setting in group and individual studies. In C. Buhler and F. Massarik (Eds.), *The Course of Human Life: A Study of Goals in the Humanistic Perspective,* pp. 27–54. New York: Springer.

Case, R. B., Heller, S. S., Case, N. B., and Moss, A. J. (1985). The Multicenter Post-Infarction Research Group: Type A behavior and survival after acute myocardial infarction. *New England Journal of Medicine,* 312, 737–41.

Cerella, J. (1985). Information processing rates in the elderly. *Psychological Bulletin,* 98, 67–83.

Cerella, J., Poon, L. W., and Fozard, J. L. (1981). Mental rotation and age reconsidered. *Journal of Gerontology,* 36, 620–24.

Charness, N. (1985). Aging and problem solving performance. In N. Charness (Ed.), *Aging and Human Performance,* pp. 225–59. Chichester, England: Wiley.

Charness, N. (1989). Age and expertise: Responding to Talland's challenge. In L. W. Poon, D. C. Rubin, and B. A. Wilson (Eds.), *Everyday Cognition in Adult and Later Life.* Cambridge, Ma.: Harvard University Press.

Chi, M.T.H. (1985). Changing conception of sources of memory development. *Human Development,* 28, 50–56.

Chiarello, C., Church, K., and Hoyer, W. J. (1985). Automatic and controlled semantic priming: Accuracy, response bias, and aging. *Journal of Gerontology,* 40, 593–600.

Chiarello, C., and Hoyer, W. J. (1988). Adult age differences in implicit and explicit memory: Time course and encoding effects. *Psychology and Aging.,* 3 (4), pp. 358–366.

Clancy, S. M., and Hoyer, W. J. (1988). Aging and skill in visual search: Dual task effects. Paper presented at the Cognitive Science Society meetings, Montreal, August 19.

Coelho, G. V., Hamburg, D. A., and Adams, J. E. (Eds.) (1974). *Coping and Adaptation.* New York: Basic Books.

Cohler, B. J. (1982). Personal narrative and life course. In P. B. Baltes and O. G. Brim, Jr. (Eds.), *Life-Span Development and Behavior.* Vol. 4, pp. 205–41. New York: Academic Press.

Conley, J. J. (1985). Longitudinal stability of personality traits: A multitrait-multimethod-multioccasion analysis. *Journal of Personality and Social Psychology,* 49, 1266–82.

Costa, P. T., and McCrae, R. R. (1978). Objective personality assessment. In M. Storandt, I. C. Siegler, and M. F. Elias (Eds.), *The Clinical Psychology of Aging,* pp. 119–42. New York: Plenum.

Costa, P. T., and McCrae, R. R. (1980a). Still stable after all these years: Personality as a key to some issues in adulthood and old age. In P. B. Baltes and O. G. Brim, Jr. (Eds.), *Life-Span Development and Behavior.* Vol. 3, pp. 65–102. New York: Academic Press.

Costa, P. T., and McCrae, R. R. (1980b). Influence of extraversion and neuroticism on subjective well-being: Happy and unhappy people. *Journal of Personality and Social Psychology,* 38, 688–78.

Costa, P. T., and McCrae, R. R. (1985). *The NEO Personality Inventory Manual*. Oddesa, Fla.: Psychological Assessment Resources, Inc.

Costa, P. T., McCrae, R. R., and Arenberg, D. (1980). Enduring dispositions in adult males. *Journal of Personality and Social Psychology*, 38, 793–800.

Craik, F.I.M. (1983). On the transfer of information from temporary to permanent memory. *Philosophical Transactions of the Royal Society of London*, B302, 341–59.

Datan, N., Rodeheaver, D., and Hughes, F. (1987). Adult development and aging. *Annual Review of Psychology*, 38, 153–80.

DeLongis, A., Coyne, J. C., Dakof, G., Folkman, S., and Lazarus, R. S. (1982). Relationship of daily hassles, uplifts, and major life events to health status. *Health Psychology*, 1, 119–36.

Dembroski, T. M., MacDougall, J. M., Williams, R. B., Haney, T. L., and Blumenthal, J. A. (1985). Components of Type A, hostility, and anger-in: Relationship to angiographic findings. *Psychosomatic Medicine*, 47, 219–33.

Epstein, S. (1983). A research paradigm for the study of personality and emotions. In M. M. Page (Ed.), *Nebraska Symposium on Motivation 1982: Personality—Current Theory and Research*, pp. 91–154. Lincoln: University of Nebraska Press.

Eriksen, C. W., Hamlin, R. M., and Breitmeyer, R. G. (1970). Temporal factors in visual perception as related to aging. *Perception and Psychophysics*, 7, 354–56.

Erikson, E. H. (1950). *Childhood and Society*. New York: W. W. Norton.

Featherman, D. L., and Lerner, R. M. (1985). Ontogenesis and sociogenesis: Problematics for theory and research about development and socialization across the life-span. *American Sociological Review*, 50, 659–76.

Felton, B. J., and Revenson, T. A. (1987). Age differences in coping with chronic illness. *Psychology and Aging*, 2, 164–70.

Finn, S. E. (1986). Stability of personality self-ratings over thirty years: Evidence for an age/cohort interaction. *Journal of Personality and Social Psychology*, 50, 813–18.

Fodor, J. A. (1983). *Modularity of Mind*. Cambridge: MIT Press.

Folkman, S., and Lazarus, R. S. (1980). An analysis of coping in a middle-aged community sample. *Journal of Health and Social Behavior*, 21, 219–39.

Folkman, S., Lazarus, R. S., Pimley, S., and Novacek, J. (1987). Age differences in stress and coping processes. *Psychology and Aging*, 2, 171–84.

Friedman, H. S., and Booth-Kewley, S. (1987). The "disease-prone personality": A meta-analytic view of the construct. *American Psychologist*, 42, 539–55.

Friedman, M., and Rosenman, R. H. (1959). Association of specific overt behavior pattern with blood and cardiovascular findings. *Journal of the American Medical Association*, 169, 1286–96.

Friedman, M., and Rosenman, R. H. (1974). *Type A Behavior and Your Heart*. New York: Alfred A. Knopf.

Funk, S. C., and Houston, B. K. (1987). A critical analysis of the hardiness scale's validity and utility. *Journal of Personality and Social Psychology*, 53, 572–78.

Glaser, R. (1984). Education and thinking: The role of knowledge. *American Psychologist*, 39, 93–104.

Gould, R. (1978). *Transformations: Growth and Change in Adult Life*. New York: Simon and Schuster.

Haan, N., Millsap, R., and Hartka, E. (1986). As time goes by: Change and stability in personality over fifty years. *Psychology and Aging,* 1, 220–32.

Hagestad, G. O., and Neugarten, B. L. (1985). Age and the life course. In R. H. Binstock and E. Shanas (Eds.), *Handbook of Aging and the Social Sciences.* 2d ed., pp. 35–61. New York: Van Nostrand Reinhold.

Hartley, A. A., and Anderson, J. W. (1983). Task complexity, problem representation, and problem-solving performance by younger and older adults. *Journal of Gerontology,* 38, 78–80.

Hasher, L., and Zacks, R. T. (1979). Automatic and effortful processes in memory. *Journal of Experimental Psychology: General,* 108, 356–88.

Haynes, S. G., Feinleib, M., and Kannel, W. B. (1980). The relationship of psychosocial factors to coronary heart disease in the Framingham Study. III. Eight-year incidence of coronary heart disease. *American Journal of Epidemiology,* 111, 37–58.

Hertzog, C. (1985). An individual differences perspective. *Research on Aging,* 7, 7–45.

Holmes, T. H., and Rahe, R. H. (1967). The Social Readjustment Rating Scale. *Journal of Psychosomatic Research,* 11, 213–18.

Hooker, K. (1985). The structure of intraindividual change in self-concept during the transition to retirement: An analysis from an interactionist perspective. Doctoral dissertation, Pennsylvania State University.

Hooker, K., Nesselroade, D. W., Nesselroade, J. R., and Lerner, R. M. (1987). The structure of intraindividual temperament in the context of mother-child dyads: *P*-technique factor analyses of short-term change. *Developmental Psychology,* 23, 332–46.

Howard, D. V. (in press). Implicit and explicit assessment of cognitive aging. In M. L. Howe and C. J. Brainerd (Eds.), *Cognitive Development in Adulthood: Progress in Cognitive Development Research.* New York: Springer-Verlag.

Howard, D. V., McAndrews, M. P., and Lasaga, M. I. (1981). Semantic priming of lexical decisions in young and old adults. *Journal of Gerontology,* 36, 707–14.

Howard, J. H., Rechnitzer, P. A., Cunningham, D. A., and Donner, A. P. (1986). Change in Type A behavior a year after retirement. *The Gerontologist,* 26, 643–49.

Hoyer, W. J. (1974). Aging as intraindividual change. *Developmental Psychology,* 10, 821–26.

Hoyer, W. J. (1985). Aging and the development of expert cognition. In T. M. Schlechter and M. P. Toglia (Eds.), *New Directions in Cognitive Science,* pp. 69–87. Norwood, N.J.: Ablex.

Hoyer, W. J. (1987). Acquisition of knowledge and decentralization of *g* in adult intellectual development. In C. Schooler and K. W. Schaie (Eds.), *Cognitive Functioning and Social Structures over the Life Course,* pp. 120–41. Norwood, N.J.: Ablex.

Hoyer, W. J., and Familant, M. E. (1987). Adult age differences in the rate of processing of expectancy information. *Cognitive Development,* 2, 57–70.

Hoyer, W. J., Rybash, J. M., and Roodin, P. A. (1988). Age-related cognitive change as a function of knowledge access. In M. L. Commons, J. D. Sinnott, F. A. Richards, and C. Armon (Eds.), *Adult Development: Comparisons and Applications of Adolescent and Adult Developmental Models,* 2. New York: Praeger.

Hull, J. G., Van Treuren, R. R., and Virnelli, S. (1987). Hardiness and health: A critique and alternative approach. *Journal of Personality and Social Psychology,* 53, 518–30.

Jacoby, L. L. (1978). On interpreting the effects of repetition: Solving a problem versus remembering a solution. *Journal of Verbal Learning and Verbal Behavior,* 17, 649–67.

Jung, C. G. (1933). *Modern Man in Search of a Soul.* New York: Harcourt Brace Jovanovich.

Kail, R., and Bisanz, J. (1982). Information processing and cognitive development. In H. W. Reese (Ed.), *Advances in Child Development.* Vol. 17, pp. 45–81. New York: Academic Press.

Karuza, J., Jr., and Zevon, M. A. (1985). Ecological validity and idiography in developmental cognitive science. In T. M. Schlechter and M. P. Toglia (Eds.), *New Directions in Cognitive Science,* pp. 88–104. Norwood, N.J.: Ablex.

Kelly, E. L. (1955). Consistency of the adult personality. *American Psychologist,* 10, 659–81.

Kenrick, D. T., and Dantchik, A. (1983). Interactionism, idiographics, and the social psychological invasion of personality. *Journal of Personality,* 51, 286–307.

Kobasa, S. C. (1979). Stressful life events, personality, and health: An inquiry into hardiness. *Journal of Personality and Social Psychology,* 37, 1–11.

Kobasa, S. C., Maddi, S. R., and Kahn, S. (1982). Hardiness and health: A prospective study. *Journal of Personality and Social Psychology,* 42, 168–77.

Kobasa, S. C., Maddi, S. R., and Zola, M. A. (1983). Type A and hardiness. *Journal of Behavioral Medicine,* 6, 41–51.

Kobasa, S. C., and Puccetti, M. C. (1983). Personality and social resources in stress resistance. *Journal of Personality and Social Psychology,* 45, 839–50.

Koplowitz, H. (1984). A projection beyond Piaget's formal-operations stage: A general system stage and a unitary stage. In M. L. Commons, F. A. Richards, and C. Armon (Eds.), *Beyond Formal Operations: Vol. 1. Late Adolescent and Adult Cognitive Development,* pp. 272–95. New York: Praeger.

Krause, N. (1987). Chronic financial strain, social support, and depressive symptoms among older adults. *Psychology and Aging,* 2, 185–92.

Labouvie, E. W. (1980). Measurement of individual differences in intraindividual changes. *Psychological Bulletin,* 88, 54–59.

Labouvie, E. W. (1982). Issues in life-span development. In B. B. Wolman (Ed.), *Handbook of Developmental Psychology,* pp. 54–62. Englewood Cliffs, N.J.: Prentice-Hall.

Labouvie-Vief, G. (1984). Logic and self-regulation from youth to maturity. In M. L. Commons, F. A. Richards, and C. Armon (Eds.), *Beyond Formal Operations: Vol. 1. Late Adolescent and Adult Cognitive Development,* pp. 158–79. New York: Praeger.

Langer, E. J., and Rodin, J. (1976). The effects of choice and enhanced personal responsibility for the aged: A field experiment in an institutional setting. *Journal of Personality and Social Psychology,* 34, 191–98.

Larson, R. (1978). Thirty years of research on the subjective well-being of older Americans. *Journal of Gerontology,* 33, 109–25.

Lawton, M. P., and Nahemow, L. (1973). Ecology and the aging process. In C. Eisdorfer and M. P. Lawton (Eds.), *The Psychology of Adult Development and Aging,* pp. 619–74. Washington, D.C.: American Psychological Association.

Lazarus, R. S., and DeLongis, A. (1983). Psychological stress and coping in aging. *American Psychologist*, 38, 245–54.

Lazarus, R. S., and Folkman, S. (1984). *Stress, Appraisal, and Coping*. New York: Springer.

Lebo, M. A., and Nesselroade, J. R. (1978). Intraindividual differences dimensions of mood change during pregnancy identified in five *P*-technique factor analyses. *Journal of Research in Personality*, 12, 205–24.

Leon, G. R., Gillum, B., Gillum, R., and Gouze, M. (1979). Personality stability and change over a thirty-year period—middle age to old age. *Journal of Consulting and Clinical Psychology*, 47, 517–24.

Levinson, D. J., with Darrow, C. N., Klein, E. B., Levinson, M. H., and McKee, B. (1978). *The Seasons of a Man's Life*. New York: Ballantine.

Light, L. L., and Singh, A. (1987). Implicit and explicit memory in young and older adults. *Journal of Experimental Psychology: Learning, Memory, and Cognition*, 13, 531–41.

Light, L. L., Zelinski, E. M., and Moore, M. (1982). Adult age differences in reasoning from new information. *Journal of Experimental Psychology: Learning, Memory, and Cognition*, 8, 435–47.

Livson, N. (1973). Developmental dimensions of personality: A life-span formulation. In P. B. Baltes and K. W. Schaie (Eds.), *Life-Span Developmental Psychology: Personality and Socialization*, pp. 97–122. New York: Academic Press.

Loevinger, J. (1976). *Ego Development*. San Francisco: Jossey-Bass.

Maas, H. S., and Kuypers, J. A. (1975). *From Thirty to Seventy*. San Francisco: Jossey-Bass.

McClelland, D. C. (1980). Motive dispositions: The merits of operant and respondent measures. In L. Wheeler (Ed.), *Review of Personality and Social Psychology*. Vol. 1, pp. 10–41. Beverly Hills, Calif.: Sage.

McCrae, R. R. (1982). Age differences in the use of coping mechanisms. *Journal of Gerontology*, 37, 454–60.

McCrae, R. R., and Costa, P. T. (1984). *Emerging Lives, Enduring Dispositions: Personality in Adulthood*. Boston: Little, Brown and Co.

McCrae, R. R., and Costa, P. T. (1987). Validation of the five-factor model of personality across instruments and observers. *Journal of Personality and Social Psychology*, 52, 81–90.

McDowd, J. M. (1986). The effects of age and extended practice on divided attention performance. *Journal of Gerontology*, 41, 764–69.

Madden, D. J. (1986). Adult age differences in the attentional capacity demands of visual search. *Cognitive Development*, 1, 335–63.

Marshall, J. C. (1984). Multiple perspectives on modularity. *Cognition*, 17, 209–42.

Matthews, K. A., and Haynes, S. G. (1986). Type A behavior pattern and coronary disease risk: Update and critical evaluation. *American Journal of Epidemiology*, 123, 923–60.

Molenaar, P.C.M. (1985). A dynamic factor model for the analysis of multivariate time series. *Psychometrika*, 50, 181–202.

Mortimer, J. T., Finch, M. D., and Kumka, D. (1982). Persistence and change in development: The multidimensional self-concept. In P. B. Baltes and O. G. Brim, Jr. (Eds.), *Life-Span Development and Behavior*. Vol. 4, pp. 263–313. New York: Academic Press.

Moscovitch, M., Winocur, G., and McLachlan, D. (1986). Memory as assessed by recognition and reading time in normal and memory-impaired people with Alzheimer's Disease and other neurological disorders. *Journal of Experimental Psychology: General,* 115, 331–47.

Nesselroade, J. R. (1977). Issues in studying developmental change in adults from a multivariate perspective. In J. E. Birren and K. W. Schaie (Eds.), *Handbook of the Psychology of Aging,* pp. 59–69. New York: Van Nostrand Reinhold.

Nesselroade, J. R. (1988). Some implications of the trait-state distinction over the life-span: The case of personality. In P. B. Baltes, D. L. Featherman, and R. M. Lerner (Eds.), *Life-Span Development and Behavior.* Vol. 8, pp. 163–89. Hillsdale, N.J.: Erlbaum.

Nesselroade, J. R., and Ford, D. H. (1985). Multivariate, replicated, single-subject designs for research on older adults: *P*-technique comes of age. *Research on Aging,* 7, 46–80.

Nesselroade, J. R., Pruchno, R., and Jacobs, A. (1986). Reliability versus stability in the measurement of psychological states: An illustration with anxiety measures. *Psychologische Beitraege,* 28, 255–64.

Neugarten, B. L. (Ed.) (1968). *Middle Age and Aging.* Chicago: University of Chicago Press.

Pearlin, L. I., Lieberman, M. A., Menaghan, E., and Mullan, J. T. (1981). The stress process. *Journal of Health and Social Behavior,* 22, 337–56.

Pearlin, L. I., and Schooler, C. (1978). The structure of coping. *Journal of Health and Social Behavior,* 19, 2–21.

Perlmutter, M. (in press). Cognitive development in life-span perspective: From description of differences to explanation of changes. In E. M. Hetherington, R. M. Lerner, and M. Perlmutter (Eds.), *Child Development in Life-Span Perspective.*

Pervin, L. A. (1983). The stasis and flow of behavior: Toward a theory of goals. In M. M. Page (Ed.), *Nebraska Symposium on Motivation 1982: Personality—Current Theory and Research,* pp. 1–53. Lincoln: University of Nebraska Press.

Plude, D. J., and Hoyer, W. J. (1981). Adult age differences in visual search as a function of stimulus mapping and processing load. *Journal of Gerontology,* 36, 598–604.

Plude, D. J., and Hoyer, W. J. (1986). Aging and the selectivity of visual information processing. *Psychology and Aging,* 1, 1–9.

Quayhagen, M. P., and Quayhagen, M. (1982). Coping with conflict: Measurement of age-related patterns. *Research on Aging,* 4, 364–77.

Rabbitt, P.M.A. (1977). Changes in problem solving ability in old age. In J. E. Birren and K. W. Schaie (Eds.), *Handbook of the Psychology of Aging,* pp. 606–25. New York: Van Nostrand Reinhold.

Rabbitt, P.M.A. (1982). Breakdown of control processes in old age. In T. M. Field, A. Huston, H. C. Quay, L. Troll, and G. Finley (Eds.), *Review of Human Development,* pp. 540–50. New York: Wiley.

Reder, L. M., Wible, C., and Martin, J. (1986). Differential memory changes with age: Exact retrieval versus plausible inference. *Journal of Experimental Psychology: Learning, Memory, and Cognition,* 12, 72–81.

Reinke, B. J., Ellicott, A. M., Harris, R. L., and Hancock, E. (1985). Timing of psychosocial changes in women's lives. *Human Development,* 28, 259–80.

Review Panel on Coronary Prone Behavior and Coronary Heart Disease (1981). Coronary prone behavior and coronary heart disease: A critical review. *Circulation*, 63, 1199–1215.

Rodin, J. (1986). Aging and health: Effects of the sense of control. *Science*, 223, 1271–76.

Rosenman, R. H., Brand, R. J., Jenkins, C. D., Friedman, M., Straus, R., and Wurm, M. (1975). Coronary heart disease in the Western Collaborative Group Study: Final follow-up experience of 8 1/2 years. *Journal of the American Medical Association*, 233, 872–77.

Rosenthal, R. (1984). *Meta-Analytic Procedures for Social Research*. Beverly Hills, Calif.: Sage.

Rowe, J. W., and Kahn, R. L. (1987). Human aging: Usual and successful. *Science*, 237, 143–49.

Runyan, W. M. (1983). Idiographic goals and methods in the study of lives. *Journal of Personality*, 51, 413–37.

Rybash, J. M., Hoyer, W. J., and Roodin, P. A. (1986). *Adult Cognition and Aging: Developmental Changes in Processing, Knowing, and Thinking*. Elmsford, N.Y.: Pergamon.

Ryff, C. D. (1984). Personality development from the inside: The subjective experience of change in adulthood and aging. In P. B. Baltes and O. G. Brim, Jr. (Eds.), *Life-Span Development and Behavior*. Vol. 6, pp. 243–79. New York: Academic Press.

Salthouse, T. A. (1984). Effects of age and skill in typing. *Journal of Experimental Psychology: General*, 113, 345–71.

Salthouse, T. A. (1985). Speed of behavior and its implications for cognition. In J. E. Birren and K. W. Schaie (Eds.), *Handbook of the Psychology of Aging*. 2d ed., pp. 400–426. New York: Van Nostrand Reinhold.

Salthouse, T. A. (1988). Initiating the formalization of theories of cognitive aging. *Psychology and Aging*, 3, 3–16.

Salthouse, T. A. (1988). The role of processing resources in cognitive aging. In M. L. Howe and C. J. Brainerd (Eds.), *Cognitive Development in Adulthood*. New York: Springer-Verlag.

Salthouse, T. A., Kausler, D. H., and Saults, J. S. (1986). Groups versus individuals as the comparison unit in cognitive aging research. *Developmental Neuropsychology*, 2, 363–72.

Schaie, K. W. (1986). Beyond calendar definitions of age, time, and cohort: The general developmental model revisited. *Developmental Review*, 6, 252–77.

Schaie, K. W., and Parham, I. A. (1976). Stability of adult personality traits: Fact or fable? *Journal of Personality and Social Psychology*, 34, 146–58.

Schulz, R. (1976). The effects of control and predictability on the psychological and physical well-being of the institutionalized aged. *Journal of Personality and Social Psychology*, 33, 563–73.

Schulz, R., and Hanusa, B. H. (1978). Long-term effects of control and predictability-enhancing interventions: Findings and ethical issues. *Journal of Personality and Social Psychology*, 36, 1194–1201.

Sekuler, R., and Ball, K. (1986). Visual localization: Age and practice. *Journal of the Optical Society of America*, 3, 864–67.

Seligman, M.E.P. (1975). *Helplessness: On Depression, Development, and Death*. San Francisco: Freeman.

Shekelle, R. B., Gale, M., and Norusis, M. (1985). Type A score (Jenkins Activity survey) and risk of recurrent coronary heart disease in the Aspirin Myocardial Infarction study. *American Journal of Cardiology,* 56, 221–25.

Sherry, D. F., and Schacter, D. L. (1987). The evolution of multiple memory systems. *Psychological Review,* 94, 439–54.

Siegler, I. C., and Costa, P. T. (1985). Health behavior relationships. In J. E. Birren and K. W. Schaie (Eds.), *Handbook of the Psychology of Aging.* 2d ed., pp. 144–66. New York: Van Nostrand Reinhold.

Siegler, I. C., George, L. K., and Okun, M. A. (1979). A cross-sequential analysis of adult personality. *Developmental Psychology,* 15, 350–51.

Siegler, I. C., Nowlin, D. B., and Blumenthal, J. A. (1980). Health and behavior: Methodological considerations for adult development and aging. In L. W. Poon (Ed.), *Aging in the 1980s: Psychological Issues,* pp. 599–612. Washington, D.C.: American Psychological Association.

Siegler, I. C., Nowlin, J. B., Blumenthal, J. A., Barefoot, J. C., Williams, R. B., Hooker, K. A., Woodbury, M. A., and Manton, K. G. (1987). The Type A behavior pattern in later life. Manuscript, Duke University Medical Center, Durham, North Carolina.

Skolnick, A. (1966). Stability and interrelationships of thematic test imagery over twenty years. *Child Development,* 37, 389–96.

Soldo, B. J. (1980). America's elderly in the 1980s. *Population Bulletin,* 35. No. 4. Washington, D.C.: Population Reference Bureau, Inc.

Spieth, W. (1965). Slowness of task performance and cardiovascular diseases. In A. T. Welford and J. E. Birren (Eds.), *Behavior, Aging, and the Nervous System.* Springfield, Ill.: Charles C. Thomas.

Sternberg, R. J. (in press). Lessons from the life-span: What theorists of intellectual development among children can learn from their counterparts studying adults. In E. M. Hetherington, R. M. Lerner, and M. Perlmutter (Eds.), *Child Development in Life-Span Perspective.*

Stevens, D. P., and Truss, C. V. (1985). Stability and change in adult personality over 12 and 20 years. *Developmental Psychology,* 21, 568–84.

Tuddenham, R. D. (1959). The consistency of personality ratings over two decades. *Genetic Psychology Monographs,* 60, 3–29.

Vaillant, G. E. (1977). *Adaptation to Life.* Boston: Little, Brown and Co.

Welford, A. T. (1958). *Ageing and Human Skill.* London: Oxford University Press.

Whitbourne, S. K. (1985). The psychological construction of the life span. In J. E. Birren and K. W. Schaie (Eds.), *Handbook of the Psychology of Aging.* 2d ed., pp. 594–618. New York: Van Nostrand Reinhold.

Wickens, C. D., Braune, R., and Stokes, A. (1987). Age differences in the speed and capacity of information processing: 1. A dual-task approach. *Psychology and Aging,* 2, 605–14.

Williams, R. B., Barefoot, J. C., Haney, T. L., Harrell, F. E., Blumenthal, J. A., Pryor, D. B., and Peterson, B. (1986). Type A behavior and angiographically documented coronary atherosclerosis in a sample of 2,289 patients. Paper presented at the annual meeting of the American Psychosomatic Society, March 20–30, Baltimore.

Williams, R. B., Haney, T. L., Lee, K. L., Kong, Y. H., Blumenthal, J. A., and

Whalen, R. F. (1980). Type A behavior, hostility, and coronary atherosclerosis. *Psychosomatic Medicine, 42,* 539–49.

Willis, S. L., and Schaie, K. W. (1986). Practical intelligence in later adulthood. In R. J. Sternberg and R. K. Wagner (Eds.), *Practical Intelligence: Origins of Competence in the Everyday World,* pp. 236–68. New York: Cambridge University Press.

Zevon, M. A., and Tellegen, A. (1982). The structure of mood change: An idiographic/ nomothetic analysis. *Journal of Personality and Social Psychology, 43,* 111–22.

4. THEORY AND RESEARCH IN SOCIAL GERONTOLOGY

Nancy J. Osgood

HISTORICAL OVERVIEW

Introduction

In their landmark chapter entitled "Scope, Concepts and Methods in the Study of Aging," published in the *Handbook of Aging and the Social Sciences,* Maddox and Wiley (1976) present an in-depth overview of the early historical development of the field of social gerontology. Maddox and Wiley focus on two major periods in the early history of the field: the earliest period in which aging and the aged were viewed as a social problem; and a later period in which a more social scientific approach to issues of aging developed.

Maddox and Wiley discuss major themes and issues that dominated thinking and research in the early 1900s. They also describe seminal works, important conferences, watershed periods, and other early events that significantly shaped the development of the field. The first section of this chapter draws heavily upon the work of Maddox and Wiley.

The Social Problem Focus

Interest in aging is quite old, but the systematic study of aging and the aged is relatively recent. It was not until the late nineteenth century that European scientists began to seriously investigate the phenomenon of aging. Increasing life expectancy and growing numbers of older persons in the population provided the initial impetus for study. Many viewed with concern, and even alarm, the implications of these and other demographic trends in western industrialized countries. The aged as a group were singled out. Social problems such as poverty, incapacity, and isolation were among those identified in this population. In the 1930s the problems of late life were being described, and the old were identified as a problem group in the United States (Maddox, 1970).

Two perspectives on social problems predominated in early studies: a social pathology perspective and a social disorganization view (Maddox and Wiley, 1976). From the social pathology perspective, social problems of the aged are explained by faults in the older individual, and the solution lies with changing older individuals themselves. In contrast, viewed from the social disorganization perspective, social problems result from breakdowns in the society and in social relationships and structures. Inequitable distribution of social resources such as income are responsible for mental breakdown in the older adult. The solution is to change the way social reality is constructed and the way social power is distributed so that conditions are more favorable to the old.

The Scientific Study of Aging

The social scientific study of aging began in the United States in the second quarter of the twentieth century. Much of the early work on aging as a social problem had already identified most of the research issues and laid the groundwork for later conceptual and theoretical development. From the early studies the following issues emerged: "the social and cultural as distinct from the biological meaning of age; age as a basis for the allocation of social roles and resources over the life span; the bases of social integration and adaptation in the later years of life; and the special methodological problems of studying time-dependent processes over the life cycle and of interpreting observed stability and change" (Maddox and Wiley, 1976, p. 3).

In his landmark work on age and sex categories Linton (1942) asserted that while age and sex are important social categories in all societies, the meanings of each vary by culture. Linton thus recognized a sociocultural dimension of age and identified age in other than purely biological terms. A few years later the Social Science Research Council published a planning report edited by Pollak (1948) identifying age as a dependent variable and noting that the meaning of "old" varies by social and cultural context. Ethnic and subcultural variations in the aging process were addressed. The basis for the study of aging as a social phenomenon was thus laid.

The first major work that identified age as a basis for the allocation of roles, power, and resources in society was *Aging and Society* by Riley and Foner (1968). In their later book, *A Sociology of Age Stratification,* Riley and colleagues (1972) developed the theory of age stratification in society, arguing that age serves as the basis for allocation of roles and resources in society. Riley et al. (1972) conceived of society as divided into various age strata, just as social stratification theorists had earlier conceived of society as divided into various strata on the basis of socioeconomic status. Society was viewed as a succession of age cohorts. This theory will be discussed in greater detail in a later section.

The ways in which older individuals are integrated into social groups and the larger society has been a major concern of researchers in the last few decades. In his important book, *Social Integration of the Aged,* Rosow (1967) examines changes in social integration of the aged in industrialized countries. Rosow identifies age segregation as the basis of social integration of the old, noting the importance of living among age peers. Rosow's research provided the framework for the social integration theory of aging, which will be discussed in greater detail in a later section of this chapter.

Many researchers have focused their attention on adaptation in late life, variously conceived of as morale, life satisfaction, or mental health. The Duke Longitudinal Studies, begun in 1955 and continuing today, have focused on biomedical, psychological, and social adaptation in middle and late life. Similarly, the Langley Porter Studies, launched in the mid 1950s at the Langley Porter Neuropsychiatric Institute at the University of California, examined causes and consequences of mental illness in the elderly (Lowenthal, 1964; Clark and Anderson, 1967).

The Kansas City Studies of Adult Life, begun in the late 1950s at the University of Chicago, also investigated adaptation in late life. The first major social theory, the disengagement theory published by Cumming and Henry in *Growing Old* (1961), grew out of the Kansas City Studies. The disengagement theory will be discussed in greater detail in a later section of this chapter.

As early as 1959 James Birren recognized the need to distinguish age differences from period (environmental) and cohort (historical/generational) differences. This methodological issue continues to be the dominant methodological issue in the field. Much current research effort is directed toward distinguishing true aging effects or developmental effects from effects related to period or cohort. Spurred by this concern, new, more sophisticated research designs and strategies of analysis have been developed in the past twenty years.

In cross-sectional studies, age and cohort effects are confounded because individuals of different ages and cohorts are surveyed at the same time. In longitudinal studies, designed to follow one or more cohorts through time taking measurements at different points in time, effects of age and period are confounded. A cross-sequential design is necessary to adequately separate age, cohort, and period effects (Busse and Maddox, 1985). For a more detailed discussion of cross-sequential analysis, the reader is referred to the following two sources: Maddox and Wiley (1976) and Schaie (1976).

Substantive Issues

Clark Tibbitts, who popularized the term *social gerontology* in the *Handbook of Social Gerontology* (1960), defined social gerontology as "an organized field of knowledge concerned with the behavioral aspects of aging in the individual, with aging as a societal phenomenon, and with the interrelationship between the two'' (p. 3). Such a definition encompasses economic and cultural facets of aging such as employment, retirement, housing, income, education, age-grading, age norms, and attitudes toward aging.

One major area of focus that dominated early research and remains important today is the demography of aging, including the size, distribution, and composition of the population. Mobility and migration patterns have also occupied the interest of social gerontologists (Tibbitts, 1960; Hauser, 1976; Longino et al., 1984; LaGreca et al., 1985).

The impact of environment on older adults, especially as it affects adjustment to aging, has also been a major concern of social gerontologists for the past several decades (Tibbitts, 1960; Lawton, 1980; Kahana, 1974; Moos, 1974). Housing and living environments have been a topic for research since social gerontology became a discipline and continue to dominate today (Tibbitts, 1960; Osgood, 1982b; Rosow, 1967; Sherman et al., 1968; Carp, 1976).

Relationships in primary groups such as family, friendship, and neighborhood groups, as well as role involvements in secondary groups such as work, church, voluntary organizations, and community and political groups, reflect social gerontologists' concern for role and status changes through successive phases of the life course (Sussman, 1976; Shanas and Streib, 1965; Lowenthal et al., 1975; Palmore, 1981). The effects of major role losses, such as the loss of the work role through retirement and the loss of the role of spouse through widowhood, on the older individual were of interest to pioneers in social gerontology and continue to be of major concern to modern researchers as well (Miller, 1965; Lopata, 1971; Blau, 1956, 1973; Atchley, 1976; Osgood, 1982a).

Most of the research issue areas identified over two decades ago by pioneers such as Clark Tibbitts, Ernest Burgess, Ethel Shanas, Gordon Streib, Wilma Donahue, Robert Binstock, and others still dominate the field today. New and different dimensions of each issue have been identified by present-day researchers and some of these will be discussed in a later section. Concern with allocation of roles and resources on the basis of age, patterns of integration and adaptation of older adults, and some of the methodological issues surrounding the age/period/cohort (APC) distinction have influenced the development of concepts and theories in the field.

THEORETICAL PERSPECTIVES

Introduction

Theory development in social gerontology is very recent. The first theory that addressed the process of adaptation to the aging process primarily from a social, rather than a biological or psychological, perspective was put forth by Cumming and Henry in 1961. Since the first social theory appeared, numerous other social theories of aging, concerned with adaptation to aging, the process of social integration of the aged, the place and role of older adults in modernized society, and various other social aspects of the aging process, have been articulated in the literature. Some theories have received limited empirical support, while others have stood the test of empirical research rather well.

Early theories, sometimes referred to as "first generation theories," were primarily concerned with the aging individual. Cumming and Henry and other early theorists attempted to explain how the older adult adjusts to major role changes of late life and how various social involvements influenced adjustment or morale. The next wave of theories, of which activity theory is a good example, were either extensions or modifications of these early theories. More recently, social theories of aging have taken a broader focus, concentrating on the environment and the society as a whole, rather than on the aging individual. These theories attempt to explain the position and behavior of older adults in various types of social and cultural environments. Dowd's exchange theory of aging and the recent school of social ecology are representative of more recent social theories of aging. At present, no "grand" theory guides research in social gerontology. Rather, many different theoretical perspectives exist side by side. Some of the major theoretical perspectives will be discussed in this section.

Disengagement Theory

The first formally stated social theory of aging is the disengagement theory found primarily in its original formulation by Cumming and Henry (1961) in *Growing Old: The Process of Disengagement*. Based on a five-year study of 275 people between the ages of fifty and ninety, who were in good health and had the minimum money needed for independence, disengagement theory referred to aging as "an inevitable mutual withdrawal or disengagement, resulting in decreased interaction between the aging person and others in the social system he belongs to" (p. 14).

Cumming and Henry discovered that older individuals gradually withdraw from social interaction and involvement in groups, organizations, and roles characteristic of middle age, and they turn their attention inward, focusing concern on the self. Disengagement was seen as an intrinsic developmental process that was biologically based, a response to declining energy and shrinking life space, both of which characterize the aging process. The theory contends that it is normal and positive for people to decrease their activity and seek more passive roles as they age. It also suggests that the individual and society mutually agree to prepare for the time when serious illness or death will cause a final disengagement. A gradual withdrawal by both the individual and society makes it possible to maintain the two in equilibrium. Thus, when death comes, the individual feels freed of societal functions and obligations, and society does not experience a severe disruption. It is also suggested that both society and the older individual derive a sense of satisfaction from this decreased involvement.

This process, which is inevitable and universal, is readily accepted by the individual and facilitates successful aging.

Theorists of disengagement were greatly influenced by the school of theory known as functionalism (or structural functionalism). Functionalism, one of the oldest sociological theories, has been used in biology, psychology, and anthropology. Employing an organic analogy, structural functionalists view society as a smoothly functioning system. Every process, institution, and configuration of roles and relationships contributes to the overall functioning of the social system, just as digestion, respiration, and other physiological processes are necessary for an organism to function.

The concept of function implies "needs" of the social system, which are fulfilled by some particular social process. Employing this type of analysis, Durkheim (1964) discussed the functions of the division of labor in society as integrative or contributing to social solidarity, and he described the four functions of religion in society as: disciplinary, cohesive, revitalizing, and euphoric (Durkheim, 1954). Talcott Parsons, the leading exponent of functionalism in U.S. sociology, first applied the theory to the process of aging in a 1960 paper and later in a brief essay written in 1963. According to Parsons, U.S. society has certain functional requirements, one of which is to have people in key positions who will be able to carry out their jobs without interruption. Therefore, disengagement of the old (who are closer to death) is a functional necessity if the society is to continue in equilibrium and satisfy the needs of the social system. Parsons also points out that our system of values emphasizes youth, newness, productivity, and materialism. Instrumental activities, such as we in the United States value, emphasize physical strength and agility and thus favor the young over the old. Parsons views disengagement as a case of freeing the old from ascriptive ties, which is a central theme in the development of advanced societies (Parsons, 1960, p. 172). Old age is described as a "consummatory" phase of life in which older individuals are free to enjoy the harvests of life without the burden of social participation and power (Parsons, 1963).

Disengagement is a functionalist theory. Disengagement is viewed as functional for society and for older individuals. The process is functional for society because (1) it eliminates the turmoil, disruption, and disequilibrium caused by the death of a fully engaged person and assures an uninterrupted continuation of the social system and an orderly transition of power from older to younger members, and (2) it opens up slots in the social and economic system for young individuals, who have more up-to-date knowledge and skills and are more dependable because they are less likely to die. The process is functional for the older individual because (1) he or she has less energy to perform major social roles and carry out activities in groups and organizations, and (2) he or she realizes that skills and capacities to function effectively are declining and death is imminent. Those individuals who achieve a new sense of equilibrium characterized by greater psychological distance, altered types of relationships, and decreased social interaction are the happiest in late life. The disengagement theory has received very little empirical support when it has been tested over the past twenty years.

Activity Theory

Although the formal statement of activity theory did not appear in the literature until after disengagement theory, previous studies conducted in the 1950s and 1960s (Havighurst and Albrecht, 1953; Kutner et al., 1956; Havighurst, 1961) had already revealed a strong positive correlation between remaining active and being happy. The basic premise of the activity theory of aging is that the older person who stays active in groups and organizations ages optimally and remains happy. The theory espouses the U.S. formula for happiness: "Keep active to remain happy!"

Activity theory, which has been called the "dominant paradigm in the field" (Decker, 1980), suggests that older individuals are essentially the same as middle-aged and younger individuals and have the same psychological and social needs: all individuals need to stay active and involved with people in social groups and organizations, to resist shrinkage of their life space and social involvement, and to find substitutes for lost roles in work, family, and community in order to maintain a sense of personal identity and positive self-concept and to maintain social support and affirmation of themselves as valuable, useful human beings. As Havighurst, Neugarten, and Tobin (1968) stated the position: "Old people are the same as middle-aged people with essentially the same psychological and social needs. . . . The older person who ages optimally is the person who stays active and manages to resist the shrinkage of his social world" (p. 161).

The activity theory has its basis within the symbolic interactionist school of sociological theory, which emphasizes the importance of social role involvement and communication with others in social groups to self-concept and personal well-being. George Herbert Mead (1934), Charles Horton Cooley (1964), and other symbolic interactionists all maintain that the self emerges, develops, and is maintained through social interaction with others. It is through communication and social discourse with others in social groups that each of us comes to know what are appropriate and inappropriate behaviors and to confirm and reaffirm our identity and image of our self. Social activity is the very core of our lives, according to symbolic interactionists.

Symbolic interactionists claim that a person's well-being is derived from participation in social groups because people are tied to groups by occupying positions in these groups and adhering to the roles that they are expected to play in group contexts. Playing roles provides for the development of personal identities through the process of role-taking, that is, of sharing the viewpoint of another. By interacting with others playing contemporary roles, one acts out and sustains an identity. When the other ceases to exist, one's identity also ceases to exist because its locus, as it were, was formed in the process of interaction between the self and the other.

Theories of symbolic interaction provide certain basic assumptions about the construction of social reality, including self-identity as it emerges in social interaction (Berger and Luckman, 1966; Blumer, 1969; McCall and Simmons, 1966). These assumptions are: (1) that identities are formulated in a complicated process of social interaction that involves symbolic definitions of the self, the other, and the situation, (2) that repeated interaction with the same other, in similar situations, results in a definite and stable self and other identities, (3) these identities are modified as the self, the other, or the definition of the situation changes, and (4) the removal of the "significant others" from interaction with the self will necessitate a reformulation of the identities in which he or she was involved.

Borrowing from the concepts and ideas of this school of thought, Lemon, Bengtson, and Peterson (1972) put forth an axiomatic statement of the activity theory: "Activity provides various role supports necessary for reaffirming one's self concept . . . .Role supports are necessary for the maintenance of a positive self concept, which in turn is associated with high life satisfaction" (p. 519).

Social Integration Theory

The next major social theory of aging to be discussed in this chapter is the social integration theory proposed by Irving Rosow (1967) and expanded upon by Nancy Osgood (1982b). The social integration theory of aging, which posits a strong positive relationship between associating with or living among age peers and morale in late life, is derived in part from the earlier theory of social integration found in the writings of the classic French sociologist, Emile Durkheim.

Durkheim's interest in social integration stems from the theoretical premise that social integration is necessary both for the maintenance of the social order and the happiness of individuals (Durkheim, 1951). In *Suicide,* Durkheim suggested that happiness depends upon one's finding a sense of meaning outside oneself that occurs only in the context of group involvement. Durkheim sought explanations for variations in the suicide rate in terms of the degree to which humans are integrated into society and the extent to which their conduct is regulated (Giddens, 1971). He maintained that high suicide rates appear with certain broad societal conditions such as malintegration and lack of social regulation. He derived two major propositions, namely (1) that the suicide rate varies inversely with the degree of integration of the group, and (2) that the suicide rate varies with the degree of normative regulation. After an examination of suicide statistics for different groups, Durkheim was able to demonstrate that Protestant countries had the highest suicide rate and Catholic countries the lowest suicide rate. He concluded that integration into family, religious, and political groups is an important deterrent to suicide.

A close examination of the concept of integration reveals that what Durkheim called integration has something to do with a person's social ties to the larger group; with that person's level of meaningful interaction with other members of the larger social group; with that person's degree of social "belongingness." The concept of integration refers to personal involvement in social groups, activities, and organizations. Persons who are deeply and intimately involved with others in various personal relationships and group activities, according to Durkheim, should be low suicide risks. Maris (1969) similarly defines integration in terms of the number of interpersonal dependency relationships in which the person is involved. Durkheim found the unmarried to have the highest rates of suicide, supporting his contention that those who are not integrated into society are at risk for suicide.

The most elaborate statement of the integration theory of aging is stated in the work of Irving Rosow (1967). Rosow's basic contention is that elderly individuals' integration into the society as a whole is seriously weakened in several respects: loss of work role and subsequent loss of economic resources, loss of spouse and friends who die, and informal age-grading that places a great distance between generations. The solution for reintegration of the nation's elderly, in Rosow's opinion, lies in age-segregated communities in which elderly individuals find a ready source of friends in age peers, as well as meaningful leisure roles and roles in various organizations. Rosow popularized the notion of "concomitant socialization" when he indicated that the most viable opportunities for the integration of older people are through informal groups among their age peers (Rosow, 1967, pp. 35–36).

According to Rosow, the integration of individuals into their society results from forces that place them within the system and govern their participation and patterned associations with others. This network of social bonds has three basic dimensions: social values, group memberships, and social roles. In other words, "people are tied into their society essentially through their beliefs, the groups that they belong to and the positions they occupy or their social roles" (Rosow, 1967, p. 162). Rosow's basic contention is that constant association with age peers or living among age peers provides the basis of social integration for older individuals. As he writes:

Density fosters the by-products of group life: consciousness of similarity; embeddedness in a bounded system; development of special group norms; role specification and restructuring; generation of group supports, including workday and emergency mutual aid and reciprocity; provision of significant reference figures and viable role models (Rosow, 1967, p. 261).

Rosow developed the social integration theory based on his empirical research. In his pioneering study of the effects of age segregation on morale, Rosow investigated the life satisfaction of elderly residents in apartment buildings in Cleveland, Ohio. He classified living environments according to the density of elderly population as Normal, Concentrated, and Dense. He found that those living in the apartments that were more densely populated with elderly residents made more friends, which he attributed to the fact that friends are made among one's age and sex peers. They also experienced a higher level of life satisfaction and housing satisfaction. He further cited the following major social gains for those living among age peers: opportunities for remarriage, new identifications and mutual support, the facilitation of transition to a new role, the generation of new activities, and more appropriate behavioral norms.

Other investigators who have turned their attention to the issue of life satisfaction and age-segregated living have found support for Rosow's social integration theory. Aldridge (1959), Michelon (1954), Seguin (1973), Sheley (1974), Bultena and Wood (1969), Sherman (1975), and Sherman et al. (1968) found high levels of morale among residents of age-segregated communities that they have studied. Comparative studies of residents and nonresidents have discovered that those living in age-segregated communities have higher levels of morale than their counterparts living in age-integrated communities.

Qualitative studies of life in age-segregated communities for the elderly have provided further support for Rosow's theory. Arlie Russell Hochschild (1973), who studied one small community, discovered sibling bonds among elderly residents and a working mutual aid society in which exchanges of services were reciprocal—"the many small, quiet factors, keeping an eye out for a friend, and sharing a good laugh" (p. 409). Further support has recently been provided by Osgood's (1982b) comparative study of life in three planned retirement communities (a mobile home community in Florida, a condominium complex in Florida, and a community of detached dwelling units in Arizona). Osgood found that in each community, a strong "sense of community" developed. Everyone felt their lives were interconnected, with a common purpose and group loyalty to the community and to each other. Residents shared a common past, present, and future. They had similar values, interests, needs, concerns, and problems. They had raised their children, gone through the years of the Great Depression, and shared other social, cultural, and historical events. At this time in their lives, they faced similar problems of rising costs and limited incomes, health and medical problems, retirement, widowhood, and the approach of death. Based on the in-depth study of life in the three communities, which differed on several important dimensions such as location, type of dwelling unit, background and characteristics of residents, and activities available, Osgood concluded that age per se served as the primary basis for the high levels of social integration found in each community.

In a similar view, Eisenstadt (1956), Merton (1957), and Messer (1967) have argued that age-concentrated environments have the potential to become normative systems for residents, alleviating role conflict by insulating the activities of residents from those members of their "role-set" who occupy different status positions. Messer claims that a physical environment that segregates older individuals serves as a buffer to the conflicting role expectations of a younger population. In such an environment, leisure pursuits become legitimate, as opposed to the work ethic accepted in the larger society. Such an orientation is much more conducive to those who find themselves retired. Bultena and Wood (1969) indeed discovered that normative attitudes of residents of such communities differed considerably from attitudes held by elderly individuals living in age-integrated communities, which they offer as support for the view that age-concentrated environments offer a source of normative attitudes to members. They attributed this fact to the abundance of role models exemplifying a positive orientation to leisure roles and the relative insulation from the work ethic.

Rose and Peterson (1965) and others have noted the development of an aged subculture, facilitated by age-segregated living. Rose and Peterson suggest that this subculture "provides a network of interrelationships and serves as a social and cultural milieu for the older individual" (p. 64). As they put it: "Not only can the potential range of social relationships be expanded, but also age-segregated living can provide socialization into, and favorable evaluation of, age-linked roles" (p. 252). They also noted the importance of shared values in facilitating the aging process.

Age Stratification of Society

The theory of age stratification put forth by Riley (1971) and Foner (1975) is less a formal theory and more a conceptual framework for examining the influence of societal processes and changes on aging and the old. Drawing heavily from early theories of social stratification of society, developed by such well-known sociologists as Karl Marx, Max Weber, and Thorstein Veblen, Riley and colleagues conceived of society as comprised of various age strata, just as many of the forefathers in sociology had previously conceived of society as comprised of various socioeconomic classes. The parallels between age stratification theory and social stratification theory are striking. In this section we will first briefly discuss the work of early social stratification theorists to provide a useful context for understanding major concepts and propositions of age stratification theory. Then, we will turn our attention to an examination of age stratification theory.

Varying definitions of social class can be found in the writings of classical sociologists such as Karl Marx and Max Weber, as well as in the works of modern-day scholars. A purely economic definition of class was put forward by Marx (1909): "The owners of mere labor-power, the owners of capital, and the landlord, whose respective sources of income are wages, profit and ground rent, in other words, wage laborers, capitalists and landlords, form the three great classes of modern society resting upon the capitalist mode of production" (p. 1031).

Marx specifically emphasized the importance of one's position in the production process in providing the crucial life experience for the individual, which, in turn, determines one's beliefs and actions. Marx's theory of the development of "class consciousness" rests on the premise that individuals similarly located in the production process will hold similar values and beliefs and will develop ready communication of ideas and group solidarity in their common struggle against those who own the means of production.

A similar but broader definition of social class can be found in the writings of Weber, a contemporary of Marx. Weber emphasized the economic nature of social class and the "market," but he also discussed personal life chances and life experiences as an element of class. Weber (1966) made a distinction between social "classes" and social "status groups." The social class one belongs to, according to Weber, is determined by whether or not one owns property. Those in the higher social class own property; those who do not own property are in the lower socioeconomic class. Accordingly, the propertied belong to the class of "rentiers" or "entrepreneurs." Weber identified "status groups" as groups differing in styles of life and social conventions. Different styles of fashion, for example, are exhibited by members of different status groups. The basic difference between "classes" and "status groups," according to Weber, is that "classes" are stratified according to their relations to the production and acquisition of goods, whereas "status groups" are stratified according to the principles of their consumption of goods as represented by special "styles of life" (p. 27).

In his classic work, *The Theory of the Leisure Class,* Veblen (1953) differentiates the leisure class in terms of social "tastes" and leisure life-styles that distinguish it from other social classes. Those in the "leisure class" engage in conspicuous consumption, enjoying fine wines and smoking materials, fox hunting, and other entertainments reserved for those who possess excess time and money.

Classes are broad social categories that, at least in part, reflect similarities in styles of life. The life-styles associated with people in the same class category include, among other things, particular orientations to manners, speech, clothing styles, education, and, in the United States, "success" (Mizruchi, 1964). All of these elements involve both reaction to and manipulation of symbols. These symbols, as used by actors in social contexts, serve as guides for the classification of individuals in class categories and, consequently, for anticipation of similar and differential group associations. There is a tendency for people with similar styles of life to participate together in both formal and informal groups, to marry one another, and to choose activities that reflect their similar value orientations.

Occupation is a major determinant of social class today. In *Sociology of Occupations and Professions,* Pavalko (1971) stresses the importance of occupational roles in linking individuals and the social structure. According to Pavalko, whose analysis is reminiscent of Durkheim's (1964) earlier writings, particularly of *The Division of Labor in Society,* working groups pattern social interactions and integrate the individual into a major social institution.

Pavalko, like Marx and Durkheim, recognizes the importance of occupation in establishing values and determining behaviors. Pavalko characterizes occupational groups as distinctive subcultures with distinct sets of norms and values that emerge, are learned, and regulate behavior within the area of work. Work is defined as a basic or central institution because it plays a pervasive role in social, economic, and other aspects of life. As many sociologists of occupation have discovered, where one works, the nature of the work tasks, its timing, the income derived, and its prestige in the eyes of others are all important aspects of work that affect the nature of life outside work.

Social class is an important concept allowing us to categorize people scientifically and to describe important aspects of their behavior in groups. We can gain valuable information about attitudinal, valuational, and behavioral differences by knowing the social class category in which people may be placed. Research has demonstrated social class differences in such varied social phenomena as childrearing practices, health status, suicide rates, religious identification, political behavior, and participation in voluntary associations, to select but a few areas of behavioral variation (Antonousky, 1967; Hollingshead and Redlich, 1958; Mizruchi, 1960; Goode, 1961; Weeks, 1943; Wilensky, 1961; Srole, 1962; Brofenbrenner, 1966; Lazarsfeld, Berelson, and Gaudet, 1944).

Drawing heavily on the concepts and ideas of social stratification theory, Riley proposed the age stratification theory of aging. As Riley (1976) stated it: "A person's activities, his attitudes toward life, his relationships to his family or to his work, his biological capacities, and his physical fitness are all conditioned by his position in the age structure of the particular society in which he lives" (p. 189).

"From this perspective age strata are seen as the link between human aging and social change" (Riley, 1976, pp. 189–90). The following types of questions are addressed by age stratification theorists: How does position in the age structure affect attitudes, behavior, and life-style? What are the effects of mobility through the age strata?

Age-grading is an important concept in this theory. People of different ages occupy different positions and roles in society; and different norms, values, attitudes, expectations, prestige, and rewards characterize the different age-graded roles. History also plays a major role in aging. Each new cohort or generation of individuals begins life at a unique point in historical time and undergoes a particular set of economic, cultural, social, and historical events that have an influence on the experiences, beliefs, values, and attitudes of that cohort. The experience of aging thus is influenced by the historical time period in which one is born and raised. A cohort is defined as "an aggregate of individuals who were born (or who entered a particular system) in the same time interval and who age together" (Riley et al., 1972, p. 9).

According to age stratification theorists, the age structure of a society is constructed from four elements: "age stratum" (an aggregate of individuals grouped by age); "age-related capacities" (contributions that can be made to society by an age group); "social role distribution" (on the basis of age); and "age-related expectations" (behavior considered suitable for a particular age group).

Two major social processes affect the rhythm and pattern of human aging:

"cohort flow" (fertility, mortality, migration, and other factors that shape the age strata) and "aging" (movement from one age strata to the next). According to Riley et al. (1972) aging is bound "by the individual's characteristics and dispositions, by the modifications of these characteristics through socialization, by the particular role sequences in which he participates, and by the particular social situations and environmental events he encounters. Hence, it follows that patterns of aging can differ, not only from one society to another and from one country to another, but also among successive cohorts in a single society" (Riley et al., 1972, p. 5).

Two processes intervene to shape various age strata: "allocation" (assigning and reassigning people of different ages to roles available in a particular society at a particular time) and "socialization" (the molding and shaping of societal members by parents, teachers, and other socialization agents who inculcate cultural norms and values). Figure 4.1 summarizes the various elements of the age stratification theory.

Modernization Theory

Modernization theory, an extension of the age stratification theory of aging just described, broadens the conceptual framework by considering crosscultural and historical comparisons of the status of the elderly. The theory, developed by Cowgill and Holmes (1972) and later revised by Cowgill (1974), described the relationship between the level of modernization in a culture and the role and status of old people. The crosscultural theory was derived from a comparison of the role and status of old people in fifteen societies that differed in degree of modernization. Briefly stated, the theory, expressed in twenty-two propositions, claimed that with increasing modernization, the status of old people declines. Modernization was defined by Cowgill (1974) as the transformation from a rural way of life based on limited technology and traditional values to an urban way of life based on scientific technology and cosmopolitan values (p. 194). "Modernization encompasses level of technology, degree of urbanization, rate of social change, and degree of westernization" (Cowgill and Holmes, 1972, p. 2). Cowgill and Holmes (1972) found modernization to be associated with later onset of old age, increased longevity, increased proportions of females and widows in the population, lower status of the aged, and decline in leadership roles, power, and influence of the aged.

In his 1974 revision Cowgill identified four major aspects of modernization that have a major effect on old people: (1) scientific technology, (2) urbanization, (3) literacy, and (4) health technology. As Cowgill (1974) explains, advanced technology results in occupational specialization and renders the knowledge and skills of old people useless.

Urbanization induces geographic mobility and tends to break up the extended family. As children move up the occupational and economic ladder and relocate,

Figure 4.1
Processes Related to Structural Elements

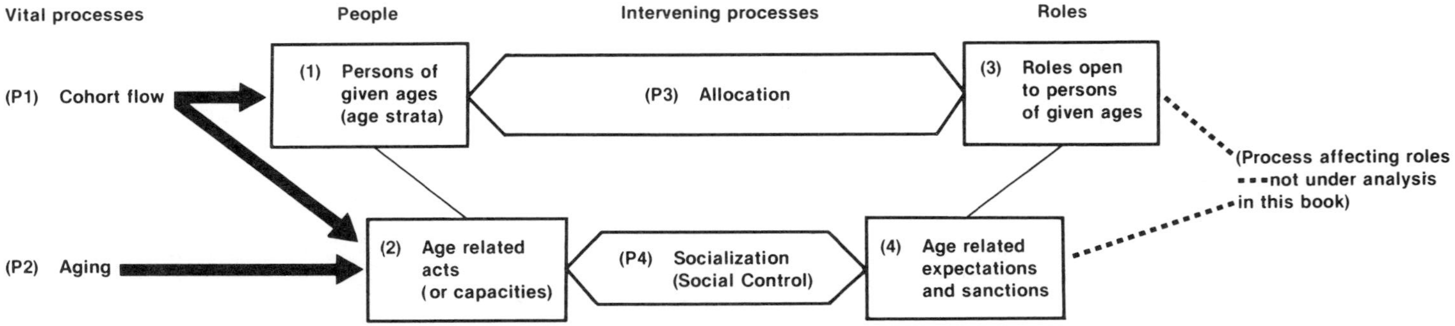

Vital processes	People	Intervening processes	Roles

(1) Persons of given ages (age strata)

(P3) Allocation

(3) Roles open to persons of given ages

(P1) Cohort flow

(2) Age related acts (or capacities)

(P4) Socialization (Social Control)

(4) Age related expectations and sanctions

(P2) Aging

(Process affecting roles not under analysis in this book)

Source: M.W. Riley, M. Johnson, and A. Foner, *Aging and Society*, Vol. 3: *A Sociology of Age Stratification*. New York: Russell Sage Foundation, Basic Books, 1972. Reprinted by permission.

older family members are left behind in lower status positions, isolated from frequent intimate social contact with children and grandchildren.

Literacy and mass education, aspects of modernization emphasized also by Lerner (1958), create a condition in which children are more literate and possess more knowledge and skill than their parents. As a result, children obtain higher status positions than their parents and often find they have nothing in common with their less-educated parents.

Advanced medical technology makes longer life a reality and creates a society in which many more older adults live longer than ever before. Increased competition for jobs and other resources heightens the resentment of the young against the old and proves to further reduce their status in the society.

The modernization theory of aging has received support in empirical studies. Palmore and Whitington (1971), who compared the social status of younger and older members of the population between 1940 and 1969 as measured on a variety of socioeconomic criteria, found that the social status of the old was considerably lower than that of the young. Similarly, Palmore and Manton (1974) found a significant inverse correlation between modernization (as determined by the gross national product, literacy rates, proportion of workers in agriculture, and other such criteria) and status of the aged in thirty-one countries studied. More recently, Maxwell and Silverman (1980) tested the theory using modernity protocols they developed for twenty-six societies using information contained in the Human Relations Area Files. They found that as societies modernized, the aged had less control of important information, were less venerated by others, and were deprived of their central importance in the affairs of daily life, relinquishing authority and control.

Exchange Theory

A relatively new theory, exchange theory, has its roots in a larger body of sociological theory called social exchange theory. Exchange theory, derived in part from the behavioral principles of reinforcement theory (Skinner, 1936) and some more modern concepts of game theory, is basically an economic theory of human behavior. The instrumental nature of interaction in dyads and small groups is viewed in terms of costs and rewards and profit maximization. Simply summarized, individuals will seek out and maintain interactive relationships that provide the greatest rewards and will avoid relationships that "cost" them more and provide fewer rewards.

Reinforcement exchange has adopted the premise of utilitarianism, as it is expressed in Skinner's psychological reinforcement (Homans, 1961, pp. 17–29). The result is a perspective stated in the positivist tradition, taking the outside point of view. Reinforcement exchange presents a model of interaction in which the controlling mechanism is the reinforcing value of a particular act.

The concepts Homans uses to develop his exchange perspective—quantity, value, rewards, costs, profit—and his propositions define interaction as a quantitative medium whereby units of behavior having rewarding value can be exchanged. Interaction for Homans is a means more than a process. It is a necessary condition to allow the exchange of rewards. Patterns resulting from this exchange are secondary to the exchange itself.

Homans' two major variables are quantity and value. Quantity is the number of units of activity that the organism emits within a given period of time, and value is the degree of positive or negative reinforcement an individual receives from another's unit of activity. Individuals enter into and remain in relationships that offer the highest quantity of valuable rewards.

Homans' "law of distributive justice," one rule of social exchange, states that "a man in an exchange relation with another will expect that the rewards of each man be proportional to his costs—the greater the rewards, the greater the costs—and that the net profits be proportional to the investments—the greater the investments, the greater the profit." Homans claims that if one's costs exceed one's rewards, or one gives more than one receives, the party giving more will become dissatisfied and the interaction will be discontinued. Alvin Gouldner's (1960) "norm of reciprocity," identified as a rule of social exchange, similarly establishes a norm of reciprocity in social relationships. Specifically, "people should help those who have helped them" (p. 17).

Extending the theory as stated by Homans, Thibaut and Kelley (1959) added the dimension of power in relationships. According to Thibaut and Kelley, an individual who can provide more and more highly valued rewards (in terms of money, position, and other "valuables") to others enjoys a more powerful position in the social relationship or social group. Power in the form of "fate control" or "behavior control" may be exerted over others by those in control of the most and best rewards. Similarly, those in control of the fewest and least valuable rewards possess the least power in relationships. "Fate control" is defined as the ability to control another's fate; "behavior control" is the ability to control another's behavior. If two people are involved in an interaction and one has total control of the money and other assets of the two, this individual in essence can control the fate of the other and probably his or her behavior as well.

Considering both the normative and psychological explanations, but not relying on one to the exclusion of the other, Blau (1964) has developed a two-phase model of social exchange. First, he assumes that the "starting mechanism" for exchange is an actor's attraction to individuals who he perceives to be rewarding to him (p. 20). The second phase involves the process and maintenance of the exchange once established. At this stage it is the "norm of reciprocity" and not reinforcement that governs and maintains exchange relationships (pp. 90–92). As used by Blau, the "norm of reciprocity" may read: an individual who supplies rewarding services to another obligates him to discharge this obligation, and the second must furnish to the first in turn.

Blau is directly concerned with individual and group power, how it is attained and used and what the results are. He defines power as "the ability of persons or groups to impose their will on others despite resistance." According to Blau's perspective, exchange processes give rise to differentiation of power because a person who commands services others need, and who is independent of their command, attains power over the others by making the satisfaction of their need contingent upon their compliance. Structural differentiation occurs along different lines in groups. Competition for scarce resources, such as material resources or superior status, leads to differential allocation of these resources according to the differential ability and regard by others that each person has. Superior status results in more power. A person's superior status is secured by (1) multiple support in the social structure, and (2) joint support by subordinates.

Once differentiated along status lines, those who are in high status positions in groups compete with each other, and others in lower positions are no longer involved in exchange transactions with these higher status persons. Blau thus lays the groundwork for a theory of how certain social groups come to possess or not possess power in society.

Building on the early work of social exchange theorists and the ideas put forth earlier by Riley and others about the age stratification of society, James Dowd (1975) has offered an exchange theory of aging. Dowd attempts to place aging within an exchange perspective. He seeks to explain the lower status and decreasing power of older adults in industrialized countries of the world as a function of the amount and value of goods and services they have to exchange. Dowd considers the old to be at the bottom of the social scale, possessing the least amount of social power of any group in society. Age strata have differential access to facilities, rewards, and goals. The old have the least control over knowledge, money, power, and other valuable resources. They possess education and skills that rapidly become obsolete in our fast-changing, complex, technologically sophisticated culture. Due to mandatory retirement policies, failing health, and various other factors, the aged become economically and socially dependent. They gradually lose power until all they may be able to offer in a social exchange is the ability to comply to the needs and wishes of others. As Dowd puts it, the old have very little of worth to exchange to obtain valued rewards. In more callous terms, those who enter into a relationship with an older adult, especially one who is sick or frail, can expect to pay a much greater cost and obtain a much lower reward than they might obtain in a relationship with a younger, healthier adult. Older people control relatively speaking a much larger share of wealth than their numbers (of course there is much variability with many who are very poor).

Social Ecology

According to Bengtson (1978), the three social-psychological needs of older people are identity, connectedness, and effectance. Connectedness refers to the need to be a part of the social setting and social group, the feeling of belonging. Effectance refers to a sense of control over one's life and one's environment and the ability to make choices and influence change. Identity is a personal sense of one's place in the world and of one's unique qualities as a human being. The environment in which the older individual lives largely determines to what extent these three needs are met. The environment also has a major impact on the physical and cognitive functioning and on his/her physical and mental health.

An individual's behavior is shaped, facilitated, or constricted by the environment (Lawton, 1980). Environments may be conducive to challenge and stimulation or they may promote relaxation. The environment can provide needed challenges, stimulation, and supports necessary for optimum functioning and positive mental health. Individuals can use the physical environment to engage in activities, accomplish tasks, compensate for loss or influence other people.

In the process of aging, alterations occur in varying degrees from one person to another and at one time or another. The need for maintenance of good health, self-determination, dignity, freedom of choice, appropriate sensory stimulation, physical activity, social interaction, meaningful activity, and social status all contribute to a sense of control and mastery within the environment, and these needs are continuous and necessary to some degree throughout life (Beck, Rawlins, and Williams, 1984).

Because the environment is such an important factor in the health and overall well-being of individuals, Kiernat (1983) has called it "the hidden modality" in rehabilitation programs. Researchers in the field of aging have demonstrated an even greater influence of the physical and social environment on the health and behavior of the elderly, who are more dependent for support on their immediate surroundings (Lawton, 1980).

The field of social ecology may be defined as "the study of the impacts of the physical and social environments of human beings" (Moos, 1974). Researches concerned with the relationship between behavior and the physical-social environment have produced a rich body of literature that confirms the importance of the physical and social environment in which individuals live and function to their optimum physical and mental health (Moos, 1976).

The field of social ecology is a relatively recent field. Theories of the impact of environment on social behavior and personal mood are among the emergent theories in social gerontology. Gubrium (1973) has been particularly concerned about the role of environment as it influences adaptation and integration in late life. He notes two environmental factors that affect the meaning old people place on events and their interaction patterns: the physical proximity of other persons and the age-homogeneity of the environment. Rosow (1967) and others earlier noted that older adults living in age-segregated environments among their own age peers had higher levels of morale than did those living in mixed-aged settings. Some older persons prefer, of course, to live in multigenerational and familial living environments, and no one type of environment is "normative" for all older persons. Indeed, a chief characteristic of older persons is their variability in almost all aspects.

Other social gerontologists operating within this theoretical framework have focused on the "fit" between person and environment. Efforts to achieve optimal functional performance require a match between the capabilities or competencies of the individuals and the demands the environment makes upon them. The less competent or able to cope one is, the greater the reliance on the environment (Kiernat, 1983). Less-competent indivduals require a more supportive environment with physical aids and supportive physical design features than do the more active and competent elderly. A proper "fit" between level of individual functioning or competence and demands and supports of the environment is necessary to assure optimum physical and mental health of the elderly.

Lawton's (1972) "environmental docility hypothesis" states that the lower the individual's capabilities relative to the environment, the more salient are the impacts of environmental demands. Thus, the less competent and more debilitated the older adult is, the greater the effect of the environment on his or her overall functioning. Lawton and Nahemow (1973) suggest that the demands or "press" of the environment must be congruent with the skills and capacities of the older individual for effective behavior to occur. Too much demand will result in fear, stress, and anxiety, whereas too little demand results in boredom, lethargy, and sensory and cognitive deprivation. Efforts to improve competence, enhance independence, and improve affective state should match the competencies of the older person with the demands of his/her environment.

Kahana (1974) presented a congruence model in which she characterized the optimal environment as one that provides maximal congruence between individual needs and environmental press. When such an optimal person-environment "fit" occurs, a high level of individual well-being is the outcome. Research findings support Kahana's model. Studies of institutionalized aged have confirmed that person-environment congruence and an institutional environment that fosters autonomy, personalized care, and social integration results in higher morale and better adjustment of residents (Coe, 1965; Kahana et al., 1980).

Lindsley (1964) and Beyer and Nierstrasz (1967) describe a "prosthetic environment," in which various physical aids and supports are available to increase mobility and prevent falls and injuries. Prosthetic environments also include sensory stimulation devices and aids to reduce disorientation, such as large calendars and reality boards with the day, month, year, and other information. A prosthetic environment is designed to compensate for various physical, cognitive, and sensory losses that are experienced by an older individual and to enhance physical and mental competence, individuality, independence, and personal autonomy.

THE NEW FRONTIER

Introduction

Many of the same concerns and issues related to the aged and aging process that were of interest to pioneers in social gerontology are still major topics of investigation today. Widowhood, retirement, housing, health care, and economic issues have remained perennial concerns. New and different dimensions of each area have emerged more recently, and, as a result, research has taken a slightly different direction. It is conceivable that in future decades many of the same substantive areas will occupy future researchers; but it is also probable that changes in longevity and life expectancy, as well as social, political, and economic currents of the future, will create a different aging experience and raise new and different concerns in each substantive area. Many changes in focus have already occurred and are being reflected in recent literature in the field. Some of these will be highlighted in this section.

Just as many issues remain the same, some new issues and concerns have recently been discovered. Problems, needs, concerns, and issues related to aging minorities and older women, in particular, have recently captured the attention of researchers and policymakers alike. Crossnational concerns and issues have also become an important area for study. Comparative studies of all types are also more prevalent today.

Suicide, alcoholism, crime, and other social and mental health problems, which received scant attention in the past, have become popular research areas in the last two decades. The role and impact of video games, computers, and other recent technological advances on aging and the aged is another very new area of investigation. Some of the more important new areas of research and interest are explored in this section.

Crossnational Concerns

One major gap in our understanding of aging is very evident. We currently know very little about the influence of social structure and the cultural contexts in which aging occurs. Anthropologists such as Linton (1942) have recognized differences in position of the old in different societies for some time. Yet, very little systematic study has focused on differences in the process of aging and the role of the aged in different cultures. As Estes (1979) points out: "Gerontological theories have tended to focus on what old people do rather than on the social conditions and policies that cause them to act as they do" (p. 11). The focus is primarily on the aging individual rather than on the larger sociocultural context in which the process of aging occurs.

In his classic study of the role of the aged in primitive societies, Simmons (1945) identified many differences in the role and position of the old in various societies of the world, ranging from the nomadic to the agricultural and more advanced. Differences in property rights, prestige and status, religious involvement, family relationships, and community activities of the old were evident in different societies. Some societies offered more opportunities for older adults to function as leaders than did others. In some societies the old held more power than they did in others. Simmons concluded, based on his monumental cross-cultural study, that the major determinant of the position and role of the aged in society is the type of society or culture. Nomadic cultures viewed the aged and aging in a different way than did agricultural societies.

The kinds of questions that we currently cannot answer, and that require good crosscultural data to answer, include the following: In what societies, and under what conditions, does conflict between generations flourish? Why? Does Gouldner's "norm of reciprocity" govern behavior between generations in all societies, or only in some? Why? What are the specific effects on the aged of social change and modernization? What is the influence of deeply rooted cultural values on the experience of being old? What are the cultural sources of old people's images of aging? How do living arrangements, family relationships, patterns of work, leisure, and retirement, and other forms of social involvement and interaction of the aged vary by culture? How does the extent and nature of suicide, alcoholism, and mental illness of the aged vary across cultures?

We have recently begun to investigate elderly suicide from a crosscultural perspective. The World Health Organization (WHO) collects and publishes suicide statistics by age groups for selected countries. A few researchers have used these statistics to analyze crosscultural differences in late-life suicide and have offered various macrocultural explanations for such differences (Altergott, 1983; Atchley, 1980; Berdes, 1978).

By conducting a national-level analysis, Atchley (1980) could show that age interacts with sociocultural context in producing suicide and that several distinct patterns exist. In many countries, suicide was strongly correlated with age (England and Wales, Germany, Austria, Switzerland, Hungary) while it was less strongly, but still positively, correlated with age in other countries (Canada, Finland, Australia, for women). Similar crosscultural analyses of data have produced more than one suicide pattern by age (see, e.g., Jedlicka, 1978 and Ruzicka, 1976).

Atchley also examined the impact of several structural conditions, such as degree of urbanization and gross national product of different countries. Age patterns in suicide for women were found highly related to economic conditions. As economic conditions improve, the strong positive correlation between age and suicide decreases in strength.

In her recent analysis of crosscultural differences in suicide rates for the old in eleven countries, Altergott (1983) found great crossnational variation in the age pattern of suicide, refuting the notion that there is anything biologically or chronologically given about the increase in suicide with age. Altergott suggests, rather, that her findings lead to questions concerning variable structural and cultural conditions that differentially impact the age and gender groups in different countries. At the present time we do not have answers to such questions. While studies have been done by the WHO on the mental and physical health of the aged in many countries, few analyses on the relationship between individual condition and risk of suicide have been conducted. This area of inquiry offers several opportunities for future research.

There is a need for crosscultural comparisons in other important areas. Until we know much more about similarities and differences in the process of aging, no "grand" theory of aging will be formulated.

Minority Aging

Until very recently the literature on aging minorities has been very sparse. Spurred by the dramatic increase in the number of minority elderly, especially Asian and Hispanic elderly, in the U.S. population, much more attention has focused on the needs and concerns of aging elderly in different minority populations (Aguirre and Bigelow, 1983; Manuel, 1982; Watson, 1986; Markides and Mindel, 1987). Some researchers have begun to investigate the differential experience of aging among different minorities and to compare the aging experience of Caucasian and non-Caucasian elderly. Research findings on depression, suicide, and other mental health problems of various minority elderly are almost nonexistent in existing literature. The National Institute of Mental Health (NIMH), recognizing this important gap in our current knowledge, recently hosted a two-day conference of experts to discuss needs, concerns, and research issues related to the minority aging experience. They have designated mental health needs of minority elderly as a major funding priority. These and other such efforts on the part of various federal agencies will ensure greater investigation of the minority elderly population and greatly increase our knowledge of this rapidly expanding segment of the elderly population. In the future we can expect to see much more attention to this group, as well as many more comparative studies.

Older Women

Until relatively recently most research has focused on males, especially research on retirement and preretirement planning. In the last two decades much more attention has been directed toward the needs and concerns of older women (Brody et al., 1983; Carp and Christensen, 1986; Matthews, 1979). Increased attention to the retirement experience of elderly females has been evident in recent publications. The most recent National White House Conference on Aging specifically singled out older women as a target group worthy of greater attention. This increased concern with the needs and problems of older women is not surprising in light of the fact that an increasingly larger proportion of the elderly population is female, many of whom are widowed. The aging experience of women will continue to occupy the interest of gerontologists in the next century. As women increasingly enter the work force, pursue advanced education, change their dating, mating, and parenting patterns, and experience a variety of other life-style changes, the aging experience of this "new breed" of American females promises to be an exciting topic of investigation.

Retirement and Leisure

In early empirical studies of retirement and leisure the focus was on the retirement experience of white males. The retirement experience of women and minorities was virtually ignored. More recently, attention has focused on the retirement and leisure experiences of women (Davidson, 1982; Paul, 1982; Block, 1982; Fox, 1977) and minorities (Watson, 1982; Kii, 1982).

Today significantly more attention is directed toward the social institution of leisure than previously. Leisure education, lifelong learning, preretirement preparation, and other such concerns have recently captured the minds and imaginations of social gerontologists (Tedrick, 1982; Kleiber, 1982; Palmore, 1982; Osgood, 1982a; Verduin and McEwen, 1984).

Most recently, McQuire (1984, 1986), Riddick et al. (1986), and others have investigated the role of video games in the lives of the elderly; and Haber (1986) and others have focused on the impact of computers and other technological advances on the elderly. These and other similar concerns will continue to guide research in the next century.

Housing and Living Environments

Social gerontologists have always been concerned with the living arrangements of older adults and with the impact of the physical and social environment on the mood, behavior, and adjustment process of older adults. Early studies examined older individuals living in their own homes in the community. Problems of poverty, isolation, and loneliness were of major concern.

In the 1950s and 1960s research emphasis shifted to the impact of life in age-segregated retirement communities, a new social development on the life satisfaction of the elderly (Hoyt, 1954; Rosow, 1967; Bultena and Wood, 1969; Jacobs, 1974; Sherman et al., 1968; Osgood, 1982b). Most investigations concluded that life in age-segregated settings is positive for older people and offers age-appropriate role models and a ready reference group, as well as greater opportunities for recreation, social interaction, and social integration. Adaptation to aging is made easier for residents of such communities (Rosow, 1967; Osgood, 1982b).

Primarily as a result of Medicare legislation passed in the 1960s, there has been a rapid proliferation of nursing homes and long-term care institutions for the elderly in the past twenty-five years. In the last decade, investigation of life in nursing homes, homes for adults, and other institutional settings has occupied a central role in the field (Sherwood, 1975; Tobin and Lieberman, 1976; Coe, 1965). Many studies have revealed depersonalization, dehumanization, demoralization, loneliness, and a myriad of other problems associated with life in institutions. Numerous studies have focused on the effect of institutional relocation (Tobin and Lieberman, 1976), many discovering increased morbidity and mortality resulting from such relocation. Others have examined the impact of size, privacy, staff-to-patient ratios, and other environmental factors on the mental health of elderly residents (Greenwald and Linn, 1971; Koncelik, 1976; Tobin, 1974). Researchers have also focused on the role of pets and plants (Cuszak and Smith, 1984), color and lighting, and various "prosthetics" (Lindsley, 1964) as they affect the aging individual living in the institutional environment.

As new and different types of housing and living arrangements emerge in future decades, the research emphasis will probably turn to these new arrangements.

Social Problems

When social gerontology was in its infancy, social problems such as poverty and isolation were the major focus of concern. Today problems such as alcoholism, drug abuse, suicide, and elderly crime dominate the scene.

The elderly have had the highest rate of suicide of all the age groups since we began to keep suicide statistics by age in this country. In spite of this fact, it was not until about ten years ago that the problem of elderly suicide received any attention in the field (Miller, 1979). In the last decade the problem of suicide in the elderly has become a major topic of research (Osgood, 1985; Osgood and McIntosh, 1986). Most recently, Osgood and Brant (1987) have completed the first large-scale national study of suicide in long-term care facilities in this country. Results of this study, although only recently published (Osgood et al., 1987–1988), have already stimulated similar research across the country. NIMH has very recently designated elderly suicide as a priority funding area. As the "babyboomers," born between 1946 and 1966, enter late life carrying with them all of the problems that they as a unique generation have experienced in young adulthood and middle age, the interest in late-life suicide will be even greater.

Like suicide, alcoholism is a major problem of the elderly (Blazer, 1982; Schuckit, 1977). Late-life alcoholism has also received limited attention until fairly recently. Recent studies reveal that alcoholism is a much more prevalent problem among more recent cohorts of elderly. If this trend of increased alcoholism continues for future cohorts of elderly, the problem of alcoholism will be more pronounced in the future. Recent studies have emphasized the role of alcoholism in late-life suicide (Blazer, 1982; Osgood, 1987), and future research may be directed toward the relationship between these two problems.

There has been a dramatic increase in the amount of crime committed by the elderly in the past twenty years. This problem cannot be ignored, and more research attention has been directed toward crime and aging in recent years (Willbanks, 1984). As the elderly become an ever-increasing segment of our population, the issue of crime in this group, especially violent crime, becomes an important concern. In the future it is probable that studies of this problem will proliferate.

Policy Issues

Policy issues of concern to pioneers in the field of social gerontology revolved around economic and health care concerns. Retirement income, pension plans, social security benefits, and poverty were of interest. Today these concerns still occupy the attention of those interested in social policy and aging, but the greater longevity and increased numbers of older individuals make such issues even more important and raise new and different concerns about how to support an ever-growing dependent population, when fewer and fewer individuals will be in the working-age population.

Health care issues have also been a major concern. Today as more and more individuals live longer and longer, concerns over how to provide needed health care and meet the ever-increasing health care demands of this group assume paramount importance. Health care and economic issues cannot be divorced. The skyrocketing costs of modern medical technology, coupled with the dramatic increase in the numbers of old and very old people in the population, have raised policy issues never before confronted. If we as a society cannot afford to meet the health care needs of everyone, whose needs should go unmet? Those of the young or the old? Advocates of euthanasia and assisted suicide, particularly for the old, sick members of the society, are gaining power. In November 1988, a bill in California, which if passed would legalize lethal injections for the terminally ill, comes up for a popular referendum vote. If the Humane Death Act passes in California, how will the elderly be affected? These and other such tough policy questions confront us as we approach the twenty-first century. Callahan (1987) in his book, *Setting Limits,* argues for rationing health care and medical technology on the basis of age, with the old receiving less.

The next century promises to offer an exciting research climate for social gerontologists. As more and more individuals live increasingly longer lives in a more complex society than previously encountered by older adults, the policy issues and research concerns become almost incomprehensible. The reader is invited to share in the excitement of discovery that awaits future generations of social gerontologists.

REFERENCES

Aguirre, B. E., and Bigelow, A. (1983). The aged in Hispanic groups. *The International Journal of Aging and Human Development, 17,* 177–201.

Aldridge, G. (1959). Informal social relationships in a retirement community. *Marriage and Family Living, 21,* 70–72.

Altergott, K. (1983). Qualities of daily life and suicide in old age: A comparative perspective. Paper presented at the annual meeting of the Gerontological Society of America, San Francisco, November 19.

Antonousky, A. (1967). Social class, life expectancy and overall mortality. *Milbank Memorial Fund, 45,* 31–73.

Atchley, R. C. (1976). *The Sociology of Retirement*. New York: Schenkman.

Atchley, R. C. (1980). Aging and suicide: Reflections on the quality of life. In S. Haynes and M. Feinleib (Eds.), *Second Conference on the Epidemiology of Aging*, pp. 141–58. Washington, D.C.: USGPO NIH Publ. No. 80–969.

Beck, C. M., Rawlins, R. P., and Williams, S. R. (Eds.) (1984). *Mental Health-Psychiatric Nursing*. St. Louis: C. V. Mosby.

Bengtson, V. L. (1978). The aged and their social needs. In E. Seymour (Ed.), *Psychosocial Needs of the Aged*. Los Angeles: The University of Southern California Press.

Berdes, C. (1978). Social services for the aged dying bereaved in international perspective. In *Suicide and Suicide Prevention*, pp. 26–41. Washington, D.C.: International Federation on Aging.

Berger, P., and Luckman, T. (1966). *The Social Construction of Reality*. Garden City, N.Y.: Anchor Books.

Beyer, G. H., and Nierstrasz, F.H.J. (1967). *Housing the Aged in Western Countries*. New York: Elsevier.

Birren, J. E. (1959). Principles of research in aging. In James E. Birren (Ed.), *Handbook of Aging and the Individual: Psychological and Biological Aspects*, pp. 3–42. Chicago: University of Chicago Press.

Blau, P. (1956). Changes in status and age identification. *American Sociological Review*, 21, 198–203.

Blau, P. (1964). *Exchange and Power in Social Life*. New York: Wiley and Sons.

Blau, P. (1973). *Old Age in a Changing Society*. New York: New Viewpoints.

Blazer, D. (1982). *Depression in Late Life*. St. Louis: C. V. Mosby.

Block, M. (1982). Professional women: Work pattern as a correlate of retirement satisfaction. In M. Szinovacz (Ed.), *Women's Retirement*, pp. 183–94. Beverly Hills, Calif.: Sage.

Blumer, H. (1969). *Symbolic Interactionism: Perspective and Method*. Englewood Cliffs, N.J.: Prentice-Hall.

Brody, E., Johnson, P. T., Fulcomer, M. C., and Lang, A. M. (1983). Women's changing roles and help to elderly parents: Attitudes of three generations of women. *Journal of Gerontology*, 38, 597–607.

Brofenbrenner, U. (1966). Socialization and social class through time and space. In R. Bendix and S. M. Lipset (Eds.), *Class, Status, and Power: Social Stratification in Comparative Perspective*, pp. 362–76. New York: Free Press.

Bultena, G., and Wood, V. (1969). The American retirement community: Bane or blessing? *Journal of Gerontology*, 24, 209–17.

Busse, E. W., and Maddox, G. L. (1985). *The Duke Longitudinal Studies of Aging 1955–1980*. New York: Springer Publishing.

Callahan, D. (1987). *Setting Limits: Medical Goals in an Aging Society*. New York: Simon and Schuster.

Carp, F. M. (1976). Housing and living environments of older people. In R. Binstock and E. Shanas (Eds.), *Handbook of Aging and the Social Sciences*, pp. 244–71. New York: Van Nostrand Reinhold.

Carp, F. M., and Christensen, D. L. (1986). Older women living alone: Technical environmental assessment of psychological well-being. *Research on Aging*, 8, 407–25.

Clark, M., and Anderson, B. G. (1967). *Culture and Aging: An Anthropological Study of Older Americans*. Springfield, Ill.: Charles C. Thomas.

Coe, R. (1965). Self-conception and institutionalization. In A. M. Rose and W. A. Peterson (Eds.), *Older People and Their Social World*. Philadelphia: F. A. Davis.

Cooley, C. H. (1964). *Human Nature and the Social Order*. New York: Schocken.

Coser, L., and Rosenberg, B. (Eds.) (1969). *Sociological Theory: A Book of Readings*. 3d ed. New York: Macmillan.

Cowgill, D. O. (1974). Aging and modernization: A revision of the theory. In J. F. Gubrium (Ed.), *Late Life: Communities and Environmental Policy,* pp. 123–46. Springfield, Ill.: Charles C. Thomas.

Cowgill, D. O., and Holmes, L. (1972). *Aging and Modernization*. New York: Appleton-Century-Crofts.

Cumming, E., and Henry, W. (1961). *Growing Old: The Process of Disengagement*. New York: Basic Books.

Cuszak, O., and Smith, E. (1984). *Pets and the Elderly: The Therapeutic Bond*. New York: Haworth Press.

Davidson, J. (1982). Issues of employment and retirement in the lives of women over age forty. In N. J. Osgood (Ed.), *Life after Work: Retirement, Leisure, Recreation and the Elderly,* pp. 95–119. New York: Praeger.

Decker, D. (1980). *Social Gerontology: An Introduction to the Dynamics of Aging*. Boston: Little, Brown and Co.

Dowd, J. (1975). Aging as exchange: A preface to theory. *Journal of Gerontology,* 30, 584–94.

Durkheim, E. (1951). *Suicide*. Translated by J. A. Spaulding. Glencoe, Ill.: The Free Press.

Durkheim, E. (1954). *The Elementary Forms of Religious Life*. New York: The Free Press.

Durkheim, E. (1964). *The Division of Labor in Society*. Translated by George Simpson. New York: The Free Press.

Eisenstadt, S. N. (1956). *From Generation to Generation*. Glencoe, Ill.: The Free Press.

Estes, C. (1979). *The Aging Enterprise*. San Francisco: Jossey-Bass.

Foner, A. (1975). Age in society: Structure and change. *American Behavioral Scientist,* 19 (2), 244–165.

Fox, J. H. (1977). Effects of retirement and former work life on women's adaptation in old age. *Journal of Gerontology,* 32, 196–202.

Giddens, A. (Ed.) (1971). *The Sociology of Suicide*. London: Frank Cass and Co., Ltd.

Goode, W. (1961). Economic factors and marital stability. *American Sociological Review,* 16, 802–29.

Gouldner, A. (1960). The norm of reciprocity: A preliminary statement. *American Sociological Review,* 25, 162–78.

Greenwald, S. R., and Linn, M. W. (1971). Intercorrelations of data on nursing homes. *The Gerontologist,* 11, 337–40.

Gubrium, J. F. (1973). *The Myth of the Golden Years: A Socio-Environmental Theory of Aging*. Springfield, Ill.: Charles C. Thomas.

Haber, P. (1986). Technology in aging. *Gerontologist,* 25, 350–57.

Hauser, P. (1976). Aging and world-wide population change. In R. Binstock and E. Shanas (Eds.), *Handbook of Aging and the Social Sciences,* pp. 58–86. New York: Van Nostrand Reinhold.

Havighurst, R. (1961). Successful aging. *Gerontologist,* 1, 8–31.

Havighurst, R., and Albrecht, R. (1953). *Older People.* New York: Longmans.

Havighurst, R., Neugarten, B., and Tobin, S. (1968). Disengagement and patterns of aging. In B. Neugarten (Ed)., *Middle Age and Aging,* pp. 161–72. Chicago: University of Chicago Press.

Hochschild, A. (1973). Community life-styles for the old. *Society,* 10.

Hollingshead, A. B., and Redlich, F. C. (1958). *Social Class and Mental Illness.* New York: John Wiley.

Homans, G. C. (1961). *Social Behavior: Its Elementary Forms.* New York: Harcourt, Brace, and World.

Hoyt, G. C. (1954). The life of the retired in a trailer park. *American Journal of Sociology,* 59, 361–70.

Jacobs, J. (1974). *Fun City: An Ethnographic Study of a Retirement Community.* New York: Holt, Rinehart and Winston.

Jedlicka, D. (1978). Suicide and adaptation to aging in more developed countries. Paper presented for the Eleventh International Congress of Gerontology, Tokyo, Japan.

Kahana, E. (1974). Matching environments to needs of the aged: A conceptual scheme. In J. Gubrium (Ed.), *Late Life: Recent Developments in the Sociology of Aging.* Springfield, Ill.: Charles C. Thomas.

Kahana, E., Liang, S., and Felton, B. (1980). Alternative models of person-environment fit: Prediction of morale in three homes for the aged. *Journal of Gerontology,* 35, 584–95.

Kiernat, J. M. (1983). Environment: The hidden modality. *Physical and Occupational Therapy in Geriatrics,* 2, 3–12.

Kii, T. (1982). Japanese American elderly. In N. J. Osgood (Ed.), *Life after Work: Retirement, Leisure, Recreation and the Elderly,* pp. 201–21. New York: Praeger.

Kleiber, D. (1982). Optimizing retirement through lifelong learning and leisure education. In N. J. Osgood (Ed.), *Life after Work: Retirement, Leisure, Recreation and the Elderly,* pp. 319–30. New York: Praeger.

Koncelik, J. A. (1976). *Designing the Open Nursing Home.* Stroudsburg, Pa.: Dowden, Hutchinson, and Ross.

Kutner, B., Fanshel, D., Langer, T., and Togo, A. (1956). *Five Hundred over Sixty: A Community Survey of Aging.* New York: Russell Sage Foundation.

LaGreca, A. J., Streib, G., and Folts, W. E. (1985). Retirement communities and their life stages. *Journal of Gerontology,* 40, 211–18.

Lawton, M. P. (1972). The dimensions of morale. In D. Kent, R. Kastenbaum, and S. Sherwood (Eds.), *Research Planning and Action for the Elderly,* pp. 144–65, New York: Behavioral Publications.

Lawton, M. P. (1980). *Environment and Aging.* Belmont, Calif.: Wadsworth.

Lawton, M. P., and Nahemow, L. (1973). Ecology and the aging process. In C. Eisdorfer and M. P. Lawton (Eds.), *The Psychology of Adult Development and Aging.* Washington, D.C.: American Psychological Association.

Lazarsfeld, P., Berelson, B., and Gaudet, H. (1944). *The People's Choice.* New York: Duell, Sloan, and Pearce.

Lemon, B. W., Bengtson, V. L., and Peterson, J. A. (1972). An exploration of the activity theory of aging: Activity types and life satisfaction among in-movers to a retirement community. *Journal of Gerontology,* 27, 511–23.

Lerner, D. (1958). *The Passing of Traditional Society: Modernizing the Middle East.* New York: The Free Press.

Lieberman, M. A. (1974). Relocation research and social policy. *Gerontologist, 23,* 266–72.

Lindsley, O. R. (1964). Geriatric behavioral prosthetics. In R. Kastenbaum (Ed.), *New Thoughts on Old Age.* New York: Springer.

Linton, R. (1942). Age and sex categories. *American Sociological Review, 7,* 589–603.

Longino, C. F., Wiseman, R., Biggar, J. C., and Flynn, C. B. (1984). Aged metropolitan-nonmetropolitan migration streams over three census decades. *Journal of Gerontology, 39,* 721–29.

Lopata, H. (1971). Widows as a minority group. *Gerontologist, 11,* 67–77.

Lowenthal, M. F. (1964). *Lives in Distress; The Paths of the Elderly to the Psychiatric Ward.* New York: Basic Books.

Lowenthal, M. F., Thurner, M., and Chiriboga, D. (1975). *Four Stages of Life: A Comparative Study of Men and Women Facing Transition.* San Francisco: Jossey-Bass.

McCall, G., and Simmons, J. L. (1966). *Identities and Interactions.* New York: The Free Press.

McQuire, F. (1984). Improving the quality of life for residents of long term care facilities through video games. *Activities, Adaptation and Aging, 6* (1), 1–7.

McQuire, F. (1986). Introduction. Computer technology and the aged. *Activities, Adaptation and Aging, 8* (1), 1–4.

Maddox, G. L. (1970). Themes and issues in sociological theories of human aging. *Human Development, 13,* 17–27.

Maddox, G. L., and Wiley, J. (1976). Scope, concepts and methods in the study of aging. In R. Binstock and E. Shanas (Eds.), *Handbook of Aging and the Social Sciences,* pp. 3–34. New York: Van Nostrand Reinhold.

Manuel, R. C. (Ed.) (1982). *Minority Aging: Sociological and Social Psychological Issues.* Westport, Conn.: Greenwood Press.

Maris, R. (1969). *Social Forces in Urban Suicide.* Homewood, Ill.: Dorsey Press.

Markides, K. S., and Mindel, H. (1987). *Aging and Ethnicity.* Newbury Park, Calif.: Sage.

Marx, K. (1909). *Capital Vol. III.* Edited by F. Engels and translated by E. Unterman. Chicago: Charles H. Kerr.

Matthews, S. H. (1979). *The Social World of Old Women: Management of Self-Identity.* Beverly Hills, Calif.: Sage.

Maxwell, R. J., and Silverman, P. (1980). Information and esteem: Cultural considerations in the treatment of the aged. In J. Hendricks, *In the Country of the Old,* pp. 3–34. Farmingdale, N.Y.: Baywood Publishing Co.

Mead, G. H. (1934). *Mind, Self, and Society.* Chicago: University of Chicago Press.

Merton, R. K. (1957). The role-set: Problems in sociological theory. *British Journal of Sociology, 8,* 106–20.

Messer, M. (1967). The possibility of an age-concentrated environment becoming a normative system. *Gerontologist, 7,* 247–51.

Michelon, L. C. (1954). The new leisure class. *American Journal of Sociology, 59,* 371–78.

Miller, M. (1979). *Suicide after Sixty: The Final Alternative.* New York: Springer.

Miller, S. (1965). The social dilemma of the aging leisure participant. In A. Rose and

W. Peterson (Eds.), *Older People and Their Social World*, pp. 79–92. Philadelphia: F. A. Davis.

Mizruchi, E. H. (1960). Social structure and anomie in a small city. *American Sociological Review*, 25, 645–54.

Mizruchi, E. H. (1964). *Success and Opportunity: A Study of Anomie*. Chicago, Ill.: Free Press.

Moos, R. (1974). *Evaluating Treatment Environments: A Social Ecological Approach*. New York: John Wiley and Sons.

Moos, R. (1976). *The Human Context: Environmental Determinants of Behavior*. New York: John Wiley and Sons.

Osgood, N. J. (Ed.) (1982a). *Life after Work: Retirement, Leisure, Recreation and the Elderly*. New York: Praeger.

Osgood, N. J. (1982b). *Senior Settlers: Social Integration in Retirement Communities*. New York: Praeger.

Osgood, N. J. (1985). *Suicide in the Elderly: A Practitioner's Guide to Diagnosis and Mental Health Intervention*. Rockville, Md.: Aspen.

Osgood, N. J. (1987). The alcohol/suicide connection in late life. *Postgraduate Medicine*, 81 (4), 379–84.

Osgood, N. J., and Brant, B. A. (1987). Suicidal behavior in long-term care facilities. Unpublished final report available through Virginia Commonwealth University.

Osgood, N. J., Brant, B. A., and Lipman, A. (1987–1988). Patterns of suicidal behavior in long-term care facilities: A preliminary report on an ongoing study. *OMEGA*, 19 (1), 59–65.

Osgood, N. J., and McIntosh, J. L. (1986). *Suicide and the Elderly: An Annotated Bibliography and Review*. Westport, Conn.: Greenwood Press.

Palmore, E. (1981). *Social Patterns in Normal Aging*. Durham, N.C.: Duke University Press.

Palmore, E. (1982). Preparation for retirement: The impact of pre-retirement programs on retirement and leisure. In N.J. Osgood (Ed.), *Life after Work: Retirement, Leisure, Recreation and the Elderly*, pp. 330–42. New York: Praeger.

Palmore, E., and Manton, K. (1974). Modernization and status of the aged: International correlations. *Journal of Gerontology*, 29, 205–10.

Palmore, E., and Whitington, F. (1971). Trends in the relative status of the aged. *Social Forces*, 50, 84–91.

Parsons, T. (1960). Toward a healthy maturity. *Journal of Health and Human Behavior*, 1, 163–73.

Parsons, T. (1963). Old age as a consummatory phase. *Gerontologist*, 3, 53–54.

Paul, C. E. (1982). Public policy and the work life of older women. In N.J. Osgood (Ed.), *Life after Work: Retirement, Leisure, Recreation and the Elderly*, pp. 119–32. New York: Praeger.

Pavalko, R. M. (1971). *Sociology of Occupations and Professions*. Itasca, Ill.: F. E. Peacock.

Pollak, O. (1948). *Social Adjustment in Old Age: A Research Planning Report*. Bulletin 59. New York: Social Science Research Council.

Riddick, C., Spector, S. G., and Drogin, E. B. (1986). The effects of videogame play on the emotional states and affiliative behavior of nursing home residents. *Activities, Adaptation, and Aging*, 8 (1), 97–105.

Riley, M. W. (1971). Social gerontology and the age stratification of society. *Gerontologist*, 11, 79–87.

Riley, M. W. (1976). Age strata in social systems. In R. Binstock and E. Shanas (Eds.), *Handbook of Aging and the Social Sciences*. New York: Van Nostrand Reinhold.

Riley, M. W., and Foner, A. (1968). *Aging and Society: An Inventory of Research Findings*. New York: Russell Sage Foundation.

Riley, M. W., Johnson, M., and Foner, A. (1972). *Aging and Society: Vol. 3, A Sociology of Age Stratification*. New York: Russell Sage Foundation, Basic Books.

Rose, A., and Peterson, W. (Eds.) (1965). *Older People and Their Social World: The Subculture of the Aged*, pp. 79–92. Philadelphia: F. A. Davis.

Rosow, I. (1967). *Social Integration of the Aged*. New York: The Free Press.

Ruzicka, T. (1976). Suicide 1950–1971. *World Health Statistics Report*, 29, 396–413.

Schaie, K. W. (1976). Quasi-experimental research design in the psychology of aging. In J. Birren and K. W. Schaie (Eds.), *The Psychology of Aging*. New York: Van Nostrand Reinhold.

Schuckit, M. A. (1977). Geriatric alcoholism and drug abuse. *Gerontologist*, 17, 168–74.

Seguin, N. M. (1973). Opportunity for peer socialization in a retirement community. *Gerontologist*, 13, 208–14.

Shanas, E., and Streib, G. (1965). *Social Structure and the Family: Generational Relations*. Englewood Cliffs, N.J.: Prentice-Hall.

Sheley, J. F. (1974). Mutuality and retirement community success. *International Journal of Aging and Human Development*, 5, 71–80.

Sherman, S. R. (1975). Patterns of contact for residents of age-segregated and age-integrated housing. *Journal of Gerontology*, 30, 103–7.

Sherman, S. R., Mangum, W. P., Dodds, S., Walkley, R. P., and Wilner, D. M. (1968). Psychological effects of retirement housing. *Gerontologist*, 8, 170–75.

Sherwood, S. (1975). *Long-Term Care: A Handbook for Researchers, Planners, and Providers*. New York: Spectrum.

Simmons, L. (1945). *The Role of the Aged in Primitive Society*. New Haven: Yale University Press.

Skinner, B. F. (1936). *Behavior of Organisms*. New York: Appleton-Century-Crofts.

Srole, L. (1962). *Mental Health in the Metropolis*. New York: McGraw-Hill.

Sussman, M. (1976). The family life of old people. In R. Binstock and E. Shanas (Eds.), *Handbook of Aging and the Social Sciences*. New York: Van Nostrand Reinhold.

Tedrick, T. (1982). Leisure competency: A goal for aging Americans in the 1980's. In N.J. Osgood (Ed.), *Life after Work: Retirement, Leisure, Recreation and the Elderly*, pp. 315–19. New York: Praeger.

Thibaut, J. W., and Kelley, H. H. (1959). *The Social Psychology of Groups*. New York: John Wiley and Sons.

Tibbitts, C. (Ed.) (1960). *Handbook of Social Gerontology*. Chicago: The University of Chicago Press.

Tobin, N. (1974). How nursing homes vary. *Gerontologist*, 14, 516–519.

Tobin, S. S., and Lieberman, M. (1976). *Last Home for the Aged*. San Francisco: Jossey-Bass.

Veblen, T. (1953). *The Theory of the Leisure Class*. New York: Mentor.

Verduin, J. R., and McEwen, D. N. (1984). *Adults and Their Leisure*. Springfield, Ill.: Charles C. Thomas.

Watson, W. (1982). Retirement and leisure among older blacks: A comparative analysis. In N. J. Osgood (Ed.), *Life after Work: Retirement, Leisure, Recreation and the Elderly,* pp. 152–71. New York: Praeger.

Watson, W. (1986). Crystal ball gazing: Notes on today's middle aged blacks with implications for their aging in the twenty-first century. *Gerontologist,* 26, 136–39.

Weber, M. (1966). Class, status and party. In R. M. Bendix and S. M. Lipset (Eds.), *Class, Status and Power: Social Stratification in Comparative Perspective.* 2d ed., pp. 21–27. New York: Free Press.

Weeks, A. (1943). Differential divorce rates by occupation. *Social Forces,* 21, 334–37.

Wilensky, H. (1961). Life cycle, work situation and participation in formal associations. In R. Kleemeier (Ed.), *Aging and Leisure,* pp. 213–42. New York: Oxford University Press.

Willbanks, W. (1984). The elderly offender: Placing the problem in perspective. In W. Willbanks and P.K.H. Kim (Eds.), *Elderly Criminals,* pp. 1–15. Lanham, Md.: University Press of America.

5. WHITHER ANTHROPOLOGICAL GERONTOLOGY?

Barbara Hornum and Anthony P. Glascock

The anthropological study of aging has largely developed as a descriptive, non-theoretical field (Keith, 1985; Nydegger, 1983; Glascock, 1982), which has primarily produced narrative accounts of the role, status, and treatment of the elderly in nonindustrial societies and among members of minority groups within the United States. Except for a few clearly theoretical works (Cowgill and Holmes, 1972; Kertzer and Keith, 1984; Amoss and Harrell, 1981), the field has been dominated by studies that do not owe their theoretical foundations to anthropology but rather to social gerontology's main disciplines—psychology and sociology. That anthropologists interested in the study of aging would look for theoretical guidance to gerontology rather than anthropology is surprising, given the fact that anthropological gerontology came of age during the 1970s and 1980s—a period of extreme theoretical ferment within anthropology.

Perhaps it is the ferment itself that led anthropological gerontologists to largely ignore theory within their own discipline and instead rely upon gerontological theories (disengagement, activity, etc.) as a focal point of their research, or perhaps it was the challenge of introducing gerontologists to the excitement of exotica that led to ignoring anthropological theory. Regardless of the cause, the fact is that a major weakness of anthropological analyses of aging is that there is a lot about aging but little about anthropology in most of the studies.

Even though few anthropologists derived their theoretical focus from their own discipline, they were still influenced, even if often indirectly, by theoretical developments within the field. It is important to chronicle this influence in order to place anthropological gerontology in its proper perspective within both anthropology and gerontology. Thus, rather than repeat previous review articles, which are readily available to the interested reader (Fry, 1988; Keith, 1985; etc.), will examine the work of anthropologists in light of theoretical developments within their field from the 1960s to the present. In this way, it will be possible to assess both the impact of the major theories that have been influential in mainstream anthropology and, at the same time, suggest where the field could benefit from a greater utilization of theoretical precepts.

It is impossible in a review of this length to consider every theory that falls under the rubric of anthropology and therefore we have been selective and have restricted ourselves to those theories that in our opinion have played and continue to play major roles in anthropological debates of the 1970s and 1980s: cultural ecology, symbolism, French structuralism, structural Marxism, practice, as well as the old standbys of structural functionalism and historical particularism (Ortner, 1984). These choices certainly open us up to the criticism of bias in selection to which we plead guilty. However, the limitations of space preclude a lengthy discussion of the relative merits or demerits of these particular theories and in fact necessitate the selection of particular figures for each theory. Thus, while we recognize the risk of simplifying complicated and often heated theoretical debates, we feel that our approach does not detract from the overall aim of the review, which is to explore the interconnections between anthropological theory and the anthropological study of aging undertaken in the United States over the past two and a half decades.

Even though, by the 1960s, historical-particularism, structural-functionalism, and the community study approach were viewed by many as "exhausted paradigms" (Ortner, 1984, p. 28), they had dominated anthropology during the previous three decades and continued to influence the anthropological study of aging during the 1970s and 1980s. This is not the appropriate forum in which to debate the strengths and weaknesses of these approaches or to trace their philosophical roots. Instead, we will briefly indicate their impact on the direction of anthropological gerontology.

Historical-particularism was the corrective anthropological response to the overexuberance of nineteenth-century cultural evolution. Its focus was shaped by Franz Boas, who more than any other individual emphasized the detailed study of individual societies using what he termed the *historical method*. Rather than the development of broad general explanatory models of human behavior, Boas argued for cautious, detailed studies that emphasized the internal development of those societies. He believed that the individual was shaped by cultural factors, transmitted via a process of learning known as enculturation. As all people, the aged are tied to the particular ethos of their group that has emerged as a result of specific historical events.

The approach led to all individuals being viewed as essentially passive reactors to culture. This particularly held true for older members of the social group who were viewed as essential sources of information on the traditional pre-contact culture rather than as dynamic contributors to the social group.

Following this perspective we find studies that are overwhelmingly descriptive, largely noncomparative, and with little theoretical discussion—characteristics of many monographs in which the elderly are portrayed as a part of life cycle analysis, as well as some of the early work in anthropological gerontology (deYoung, 1958; Spencer, 1965). Spencer's study of the Samburu provides an intriguing picture of a gerontocracy but does not tie this system to a wider theoretical discussion.

The other main theoretical perspective within anthropology during the first half of the twentieth century was structural-functionalism, which has its recent roots in the work of the nineteenth-century sociologist Emile Durkheim. Durkheim placed emphasis on what he termed "social solidarity"—the cohesive nature of social facts which function to maintain the social group. A. R. Radcliffe-Brown, working in England during the 1920s and 1930s, expanded upon Durkheim's views and placed emphasis on the social structure and institutions rather than "social facts." Thus, "a social system (the total social structure of a society together with the totality of social usages in which that structure appears and on which it depends for its continued existence) has a certain kind of unity, which we may speak of as a functional unity. We may define it as a condition in which all parts of the social system work together with a sufficient degree of harmony or internal consistency, i.e., without producing persistent conflicts which can neither be resolved nor regulated" (Radcliffe-Brown, 1952, p. 181).

From this perspective, structures are seen as being the determinants of human behavior; people act in a certain manner because they are members of specific structures—lineages, clans, age sets, etc.—and since these structures must function to maintain the social structure, there is a harmony within the social group with all the parts meshing together in an orderly fashion. The result of this emphasis on the functioning of structures is a static synchronic view of human behavior in which the analysis of individual behavior and historical or evolutionary process is absent. Individual behavior is determined by structure, and the process that is important for study is the recurrent process of structure continually seeking homeostasis.

The influence of structural-functionalism on the anthropological study of aging is perhaps best seen in the works on so-called gerontocracies and age grade systems (Hamer, 1972; Eisenstadt, 1956). In these studies the interrelation between and within the different age groupings is viewed as being beneficial to the maintenance of the society. "On the one hand the structure provides inequality between young and old men, but generational disparity is balanced by equality within generations" (Hamer, 1972, p. 27). Individuals of all ages are portrayed as members of "age groupings" that largely determine their behavior.

The third area of anthropological theory that influenced the development of anthropological gerontology was the work of Robert Redfield. Redfield placed emphasis on the distinctions between what he called folk societies and urban societies. The folk society was small, somewhat isolated, and the people in it were bound together by shared and implicit convictions about life. The urban society is based on a technical order. In it people were tied to one another from mutual usefulness, deliberate coercion, or from necessity and expedience. The implications of Redfield's ideal types for the analysis of the lives of the elderly appear to us to have contributed to the view, often held by nonanthropologists, of some ideal or mythic golden age for those who grow old in folk societies, as opposed to the isolation and alienation of the elderly in urban-industrial societies. Indeed, to a large extent many of the studies of the impact of modernization on the roles and statuses of the elderly help to perpetuate this. These studies often overlooked the problems faced by the elderly when subsistence economies experienced food shortages (Glascock, 1982). Yet even those who found negative impacts from industrialization, urbanization, and Westernization have recognized that comparative data support more complex analyses that recognize and include broader values, whether religious, political, or philosophical, that can mediate the results of modernization (Clark and Anderson, 1967; Holmes, 1983; Vatuk, 1980).

Cultural ecology dominated theoretical discussions within anthropology during the 1960s and 1970s. It, or its two close relatives—cultural materialism and general systems theory—came to represent, for many anthropolgists, a way to make the discipline more rigorous and scientific; a way to overcome accusations that anthropology was "soft," "fuzzy," and "vague"; a way to move the discipline beyond the description of exotic cultural behavior.

Cultural ecology has its roots in the work of the classic evolutionists of the nineteenth century and played a central part in the work of Edmund Tylor and Lewis Henry Morgan. By the beginning of the twentieth century, evolutionalism was outside of the mainstream of anthropology and remained so until its reincarnation in the work of Leslie White during the 1940s. It was White (1943, 1959) who resurrected the concepts of technology, energy, and evolution and once again included them in anthropological dialogue. It remained, however, for Julian Steward (1953, 1955) to introduce the environment and adaptation into the discussion. The ensuing debate between White and Steward as to the appropriate level of analysis ended with the general conclusion that both the universal evolutionary trends and the specific results of these trends as reflected in particular societies had to be studied (Sahlins and Service, 1960).

By the mid 1970s the proponents of the ecological perspective had developed a view of human culture that placed emphasis on the extraction of energy from the environment through the creation of specific social institutions suitable for particular environments. Since the environment never remains constant, these human social systems had to change, which in turn resulted in cultural evolution on both a specific and general level.

The research spawned from this perspective focused on the examination of concrete aspects of the relationship between the environment and social institutions: calorie intake in the Kalahari (Lee, 1969); pig-keeping in New Guinea (Rappaport, 1967); sacred cows in India (Harris, 1969); the destruction of property on the Northwest Coast (Piddocke, 1965). These studies were a valuable component of the theoretical discussions of the 1960s and 1970s as they established the central position of the environment in the study of human behavior, as well as a more systematic and quantitative methodology within anthropological research. However, by the 1980s a dissatisfaction with the explanatory power of cultural ecology had become widespread. A growing number of anthropologists had begun to view cultural ecology as only functionalism with an environmental component welded on. Thus, cultural ecology was subject to the same criticism as classical functionalism: it is a purely mechanical approach that reifies structure while producing "theory" that is often more tautological than explanatory. Including the environment in the analysis of human social institutions extended functionalism beyond its more traditional perspective, but it was still functionalism. Its focus was still on "how social and cultural forms function to maintain an existing relationship with the environment" (Ortner, 1984, p. 133).

The cultural ecological perspective has influenced the anthropological study of aging from its beginning. Leo Simmons' *The Role of the Aged in Primitive Society* is perhaps the first example of not only the anthropological study of the aged, but also the application of ecological functionalism to this subject area. In this work Simmons views the environment as one of three major groupings of traits that determine the type of treatment directed toward the elderly. Simmons punctuated his extensive ethnographic illustrations with succinct reports of his statistical findings, e.g., "under statistical analysis, extremes of climate, such as severe cold and aridity, appear to have exercised a reducing influence on homage accorded to both aged men and women" (Simmons, 1945, p. 79). As he had stated, "Communalism thus appears to have developed more readily under hard and difficult circumstances which jeopardized group security and even existence than in environments characterized by comfort and plenty" (Simmons, 1945, p. 33).

This approach, though, led Simmons to an analysis that is perhaps the clearest example of ecological functionalism found in anthropological gerontology. The role and concomitant treatment of the aged are determined by a series of environmental and social forces that impact individuals within societies. The result is a functional model of society in which the elderly are only one part in a complex web of interrelated components that function to maintain the society. Thus the elderly reach a point in almost all societies when further usefulness appears to be over, and the (old person) is regarded as a living liability. "All societies differentiate between old age and this final pathetic plight. Some do something positive about it. Others wait for nature to do it or perhaps assist nature in doing it" (Simmons, 1960, p. 87). Thus, the elderly play their final part within society: they are removed so that the society can function better.

Simmons has been criticized for producing a work that is methodologically simplistic and theoretically sterile but these criticisms ignore the true significance of his work: it not only drew attention to the role, status, and treatment of the elderly in nonindustrial societies but also established a framework in which other analyses could be placed, as well as producing a series of ecologically based hypotheses that could be tested with ethnographic data. Unfortunately, the ecological aspects of Simmons' work were ignored for over twenty years. It was not until the 1960s that the impact of the environment on the elderly was examined in anything approaching a systematic manner. D. Lee Guemple's (1969) study of the Qiqiktamiut Eskimo of the Belcher Islands is an example of the analysis of the relationship between the environment and the role, status, and treatment of the elderly. Guemple (1983, p. 25) found that the demanding nature of hunting and living in the harsh environment of the Belcher Islands resulted in many physical impairments among both males and females and forced "retirements" at an early age. Although Eskimo attempted to delay the onset of old age and the resultant dependency on younger members of the social group through "renewal ceremonies" and the control of property, "at the point when the elderly become a drain on the resources of the group of the community, the practical bent of the Eskimo asserts itself forcefully . . . [and] . . . the old people are done away with" (Guemple, 1969, p. 69). Once again, the functional aspects of the ecological approach are emphasized: the survival of the group necessitates the killing/abandonment of the elderly.

This functional explanation for the treatment of the elderly is given a more clearly ecological emphasis in the work of a number of anthropologists in the late 1970s and early 1980s. Pamela Amoss and Stevan Harrell, more than others who studied aging from this perspective, placed emphasis on the need of the elderly to adapt to the ever-changing natural environment. To them (Amoss and Harrell, 1981, p. 5), the survival of the elderly is dependent upon the "degree of control old people maintain over resources . . . [and] . . . the balance between the costs old people represent to the group and the contributions they make." This approach can, and often does, lead to a largely mechanical cost/benefit analysis in which the role, status, and treatment of the elderly are nothing more than that which is necessary to maintain the society's existing relationship with the environment. However, such analyses, although few in number within anthropological gerontology, place the emphasis where it is needed—on the explanation of aging and the elderly within the context of anthropological theory— thus allowing for "age" to be considered as a critical variable in the study of cultural process.

In the interest of space and simplification and recognizing the importance to symbolic anthropology of individuals like David Schneider and Mary Douglas, we will be looking at the approaches of Clifford Geertz and Victor Turner, as these appear to typify two related yet also divergent orientations to the interplay of symbols and behavior.

Clifford Geertz, in *The Interpretation of Cultures* (1973) and in "On the Nature of Anthropological Understanding" (1975), discusses the use of symbols as the locus of culture, especially nonmaterial culture, e.g., worldview, values, attitudes. In other words, Geertz sees symbols as the shapers of how social actors think, perceive, and feel about the world in which they must act. His emphasis further is on how the use of symbols by a particular group defines for that group their social relationships and also, at the level of the individual, his sense of self. In addition, by looking at culture from the frame of reference of the actor and thereby studying culture not as an abstraction, but as a mechanism through which people try to understand and behave with some ability to control their lives, Geertz asks that anthropologists try to look at the behavior of particular groups from the inside out. This is referred to as the "emic" perspective. Victor Turner, in contrast, in *The Forest of Symbols* (1967) and in *The Ritual Process* (1969), believes that the use of internal categories should be balanced by an external analytic view brought to bear on the data in terms of the development of scientific or at least objective categories constructed by the trained anthropological observer. As a consequence of his intellectual ties to British social anthropology and figures like Max Gluckman, Turner was interested in symbols as vehicles for achieving social transformations. There is a clear concern in his work with how symbols can actively effect the processes and not just the construction of social activity. Another important element in his work explores the use of symbols to help construct and maintain social ties that could override the conflict he believed inherent in most social situations.

Although there are strengths and weaknesses in both these approaches and in symbolic anthropology in general, we cannot discuss these here. At this point we will be looking at the ways in which the work of Geertz and Turner has influenced the establishment of some general categories in the anthropological study of aging and subsequently providing specific instances of these.

Barbara Myerhoff, in her (1984) article, "Rites and Signs of Ripening: The Intertwining of Ritual, Time and Growing Older," discusses both the advantages and disadvantages of the paucity of rituals for the latter part of life. The absence of socially acceptable symbols for different phases of aging except for retirements and funerals leaves the elderly person without a sense of what society expects and, more germane, without guidelines to follow except for those that they create in individual isolation. As she states, "Ritual is far more than merely expressive or communicative. It can be an active agent of change, of society, by altering the consciousness of its members. Ritual allows us to perform our thoughts, inhabit the invisible worlds of our imaginings, and experience them as real in the structures that we create for them. In the subjective mood that ritual creates, the moral order is seen from a new perspective. Conformity or questioning may result" (Myerhoff, 1984, p. 316). It seems to us that this is a clear restatement of Geertz' approach, although Myerhoff does not directly acknowledge this.

Yet another aspect of Geertzian symbolic anthropology is his focus on studying cultural events from the frame of reference of the actor. Perhaps this more than anything else has influenced the presentation of qualitatively and emically oriented views of the aging experience. *Number Our Days* (1979) by Barbara Myerhoff chronicles the life of elderly Jews in Southern California. It is a beautifully written book, in which the elderly themselves define their world and their experiences in that world. In terms of the overt use of anthropological theory, however, Myerhoff turns to Victor Turner to analyze some of the sociocultural dramas of her respondents' lives. They used symbols, myths, and rituals to sustain the collective life they had established, to restore order and balance, to reintegrate individuals or factions, to affirm cherished and unquestioned beliefs.

Similar studies by Becker (1983) on the experiences of the deaf elderly, by Kayser-Jones (1981) comparing institutionalized elderly in Scotland and the United States, by Francis (1984) looking at the life satisfaction of older people in Leeds, England, and Cleveland, Ohio, and by Vesperi (1986) in her study of life in St. Petersburg, Florida, use this same theoretical perspective in their presentation of their ethnographic data, even when no explicit mention is made nor is theory testing done.

Those studies of the elderly that explore cultural themes and values as cognitive maps used by the older individual and by those with whom they interact also seem to us to be drawing from symbolic anthropology as well. In "Japan: The After Years" (1972), David Plath discusses the conflicting themes of *obasute* or "discarding granny" and the Confucian ethic of honoring the aged. What he is able to do is to empirically test the power of cognitively based beliefs as he demonstrates that even some of the older Japanese who are living with a son may feel depressed and obsolete because of the embedding of *obasute* and the fears it generates about being decrepit and therefore unworthy. That there is ambivalence about being old in Japanese society is also traced by Plath to cognitive concepts of cyclical time clashing with the linear reality of age-cohorts.

Although very different from Geertz and Turner in the approach to studying cognition, Claude Levi-Strauss does have some concern with cognitive processes. His view of structuralism as articulated in *Structural Anthropology* (1963) and in *The Elementary Structures of Kinship* (1969) was that there were deep and innate structures of a psychobiological nature that were universal to all human beings. It is not easy to probe these structures as they are hidden beneath behavioral overlays that vary from culture to culture. Levi-Strauss believes that myth, art, and language can be used to help uncover these deeply embedded universals. Further, he feels that there is a universal pressure for classification, which manifests itself in logically constructed binary opposites. In looking at Levi-Strauss' work it is apparent that while he has little interest in explaining the surface differences and cultural variation, he does not preclude the legitimacy of adaptive or environmental explanations for them. While much of his work and his search for universal structures have had little impact on aging studies, other aspects of his thinking appear to have exerted some influence. He feels that it is inevitable for people to make distinctions between self and other, and he draws on Mauss' work on exchange and reciprocity to analyze kinship relations. As we shall demonstrate, these concepts have applicability to studies of kin and non-kin networking that often appear in anthropological assessments of older people.

In reviewing the various anthropological studies of older people, whether in small, traditional societies or in large, urban, industrial ones, it is clear that at some point there will be discussion of the roles and statuses of the elderly in relation to others, kin and non-kin and, particularly, on the types of bonds developed over long periods of time that serve as "certificates of deposit" that the elderly can cash when the need arises. There is little question of this when the old are the valued repositories of knowledge as in the study done by Biesele and Howell (1981) on the Kung hunter-gatherers. Others like Cool and McCabe (1983) and Harrell (1981) have also explored networking that grows out of long-term relationships of exchange and reciprocity to partially account for the easier transition of women as they age when compared to men. In these societies many of the reciprocal relationships of women cut across the generations, whereas male networking is largely dependent on the relations between male age-mates. This leaves older men with a diminishing pool from which to draw.

Perhaps one of the most useful studies demonstrating the necessity for durable personal ties is Charlotte Ikels' "The Coming of Age in Chinese Society: Traditional Patterns and Contemporary Hong Kong" (1980). In this study, Ikels analyzes the differences in social structures, values, and personal relationships between the traditional village, the premodern cities, and modern Hong Kong. In the traditional village there were strong societal values that motivated people to support the elderly. These included practical economic considerations and supernatural sanctions, as well as public opinion. The kin group was responsible for a continuum of care, and the older person was able to benefit from their earlier input. The premodern cities shared the same values but did not provide opportunities for the same closeness. People who had migrated to these cities in their youth remigrated and retired to the villages of their earlier life. Those who did not do so were only secure if they had families that also lived in the city. Failing that, they were in difficulty unless they had long-term relationships with coworkers and/or employers and could use those relationships when they required various types of assistance. In the modern city of Hong Kong the situation and structure of life is very different. The problems of anonymity, of rapid social change, and of increased difficulty in moving across busy streets to get to shops may present new hazards to the elderly that are not overcome by various bureaucratically organized provisions for monetary or other assistance. Ikels found that here, too, the elderly have little choice but to follow the traditional strategies of reliance on personal ties. Thus networking and its importance for reciprocity and for all types of exchanges seems to be a consistent thread despite structural variation and could be directly used to validate the thinking of Mauss and of Levi-Strauss.

Another type of structural analysis appears in what has been called structural Marxism, which differs from other Marxist-derived theories. It developed chiefly in England and France in the 1970s. Ortner (1984) sees structural Marxism as the only such theory to develop entirely within anthropology. As typified by the writings of Jonathan Friedman in "Marxism, Structuralism, and Vulgar Materialism" (1974) and in "Tribes, States and Transformations" (1975), and the work of Maurice Bloch in "The Long Term and the Short Term: The Economic and Political Significance of the Morality of Kinship'' (1974), structural Marxism sees culturally determining factors residing in the structures of social relations. It posits that it is the social relations involving the modes of production, rather than these modes themselves, that are the critical factors influencing the ways people perceive of and deal with each other. Thus cultural beliefs, values, and the like are important because they are transformed into ideology, which in turn serves to legitimate the social order and conceal aspects of inequality. Kinship, marriage, exchange, and domestic organization are included as important systemic/structural mechanisms, and the analyses done on patterns of social relations have had influence on the establishment of categories for studying the social positions of the elderly, e.g., gerontocracy.

As indicated above, structural Marxism explores the social relationships that grow out of the modes of production. Implicitly rather than explicitly this appears to have affected the various studies of resource control and how this in turn shapes the position of the elderly vis-à-vis other segments of a given population. Studies like Foner and Kertzer's (1978), which looked at role transition and change in the context of age-stratification, examine how age-cohorts may vie with one another for prestige and control when transitions actually involve or threaten to involve changes in the distribution of social rewards. While societies can ease or moderate the conflicts and tensions that ensue, these are seen as inherent. Foner and Kertzer do not debate the accuracy of structural Marxism as a theoretical model for social interaction, but they do draw analogous conclusions to Marxist theory: "Just as Marx looked for inherent sources of conflict in the class system and saw class conflicts as a basis of change in the class structure, we propose that age conflicts and tensions are intrinsic to transition processes and that these conflicts are likely to be a source of change in the age systems'' (1978, p. 1102).

A more direct use of structural Marxism as an analytic framework comes from Hendricks' assessment of modernization theory in his ''The Elderly in Society: Beyond Modernization'' (1982), in which he critiques the early studies of modernization because of their use of structural-functional analysis. These studies posited some premodern ''golden age'' for the elderly, an age destroyed by modernization that displaced the important and traditional ties across different generations. Hendricks feels that this type of study overlooked premodern stratification. The advantage he perceives in the use of structural Marxism is that it explores the relationships of capitalism on the changing structure of elites, including discussions of how different models of capitalism themselves vary in the types and severity of the changes in status for the elderly.

Finally, differentiated social structure and its vital part in shaping what happens to older people in the modern, industrial, capitalist state is summarized by J. J. Dowd in his 1980 book, *Stratification among the Aged,* when he states:

Hidden among all of the statistics and accounts of the problems faced by old people in modern society is the simple fact that some old people live fairly well while others face certain impoverishment. This fact has nothing to do with individual skills, activities, personality attributes, or other personal qualities; rather it has to do with social structure. By social structure I mean division of the American economy into sectors: one sector is highly organized and characterized by high wages and pension systems, and the other is marked by low wages and few, if any, fringe benefits. The differences between economic sectors do not end with income but include differences between pension plans and health insurance benefits; thus a worker's life is affected by sector placement, even after retirement (Dowd, 1980, p. 75).

Those anthropologists studying interest groups, ethnic groups, and preretirement behavior at the individual level present a view of the behavior of the elderly as far less passive.

The set of theories described as *practice* by Ortner (1984) provide a theoretical model where the individual is perceived as holding a more active role in interaction with the social system than that accorded by any of the structural models. Accordingly, it draws on Weber as well as Marx, on the interactionists as heavily as the structural-functionalists. Critical works that have helped to shape this model include Kapferer's 1976 volume, *Transaction and Meaning: Directions in the Anthropology of Exchange and Human Behavior,* Bourdieu's book, *Outline of a Theory of Practice* (1978), and Geertz' 1980 article, "Blurred Genres: The Refiguration of Social Thought." Although there are other important contributions, including some with variations from those mentioned, we shall focus on two aspects of practice theory that appear to us to be most relevant for studies of the elderly. The first aspect involves a recognition that while the individual has some impact on the system, the latter is a reality and must be understood as such especially in terms of systemic development and modification. The second aspect looks at interaction in terms of roles and statuses seen as linked to an almost inevitable social asymmetry. Many of the studies of older people living within extant communities like Vesperi's (1986) *City of Green Benches,* whether deliberately or not, appear to involve practice theory as they look at how the elderly try to cope with situationally presented difficulties. Indeed, assessments of communities with large numbers of older people may provide opportunities for looking at both asymmetrical relationships as well as at patterns of balanced reciprocity (Hornum, 1983).

Growing Old in Silence: Deaf People in Old Age, Gaylene Becker's 1983 study of the aged deaf in the San Francisco Bay area, draws on symbolic and cognitive anthropology but also clearly illustrates how specific groups may play an active role in manipulating their social environment. Her research, like that of Francis (1984), demonstrates that a combination of peer support and an active role in the decision-making processes that affect their environment enhances the prospects for increased life satisfaction and actual living situations. In the concluding paragraph of her book Becker states:

When the social system no longer enforces obligations to elders, or indeed even recognizes obligations, disequilibrium is established, thus reducing the aging individual's position in the social system to a marginal one similar to that of the disabled. In order to maintain a toehold in the social system, the individual must negotiate a position in society for himself or herself, using all the resources at his or her disposal. Whether this position is in an age-graded community, in an ethnic group, or in a social network made up of family and friends is irrelevant. What is of crucial importance is that the individual exchange something of cultural significance, mutually valued by young and old, since cultural continuity is the framework on which all people build their lives. (P. 128)

Whether consciously or not, then, many of the elderly are able to realistically appraise the system in which they live and proceed to make appropriate modifications to that system. They are also able to draw upon various exchange and reciprocal networks.

There is little doubt that the small but growing number of anthropological gerontologists have produced excellent work in chronicling the lives and social experiences of the elderly in different societies around the world. This has contributed a comparative component to gerontology that allows researchers and care-givers to gain a greater appreciation of which aspects of aging are universal and which are culture specific—an understanding which should prove to be useful in terms of social programs and policies. Certainly, it is important to keep in mind that there are limitations to the comparison of a study of a single, small, Eskimo community undertaken by a lone anthropologist with a demographic survey of a European population of over 100 million (Townsend, 1964, p. 36). However, Townsend's caution, although relevant for all gerontologists, does not lessen the importance of the comparative framework that anthropology offers to the field of gerontology. An equally important contribution of the anthropological perspective to gerontology is the holistic approach to data collection and analysis. From this perspective, the elderly are viewed as part of a larger sociocultural system and neither as a detached or isolated segment of a population, nor as a bundle of medical or social problems.

It appears, however, that as anthropological gerontologists work to become part of mainstream gerontology they are losing this theoretical relationship with general anthropology. In reviewing a large, if not exhaustive, amount of the research conducted by anthropological gerontologists over the past three decades, it appears that the vast majority of the studies are not based upon any specific anthropological theory. In particular, there seem to be few explicit attempts to integrate the gerontological findings into anthropological issues and concerns. It is interesting that in the one recent exception to this, the edited volume by Kertzer and Keith, the majority of contributors have not actually conducted research on aging.

This situation is particularly intriguing because, as stated in our introduction, many anthropological gerontologists do test theories derived from the other disciplines that constitute gerontology, primarily psychology and sociology. We do not mean to imply that this is not valuable, for it is. In fact, testing the crosscultural validity of these various theories derived from sociological and/or psychological research has expanded the general understanding of the aging process. Yet this does increase the possible separation of anthropological gerontologists from the very discipline that has given them intellectual and methodological life.

Why has this occurred? It could be a construct of the very nature of gerontology itself as an applied and multidisciplinary area, dominated, however, by medical and health practitioners. As a result, there is a perception among anthropologists, perhaps, that since they are presenting information to nonanthropologists they have to make it understandable and the use of existing gerontological theory is one way of accomplishing this. Additionally, anthropological gerontologists may also perceive themselves as latecomers and outsiders, people with important things to say but with a need to gain credibility with their listeners, credibility that can be attained only through some degree of deanthropologization.

Other factors may stem from the nature of the relationship of mainstream anthropology to its more applied areas, of which anthropological gerontology is one. Some anthropological gerontologists work in multidisciplinary teams in their research and in urban-industrial societies. This takes them farther away from the traditional theoretical and methodological focus of anthropology. It is increasingly difficult for many anthropological gerontologists to be classified as Africanists, Asianists, etc., since even those with area specialization in their initial research begin to focus on the elderly across tribal or national boundaries. Whether correct or not, there does seem to be some perception that this type of work is not as anthropologically valid as the more standard ethnographic research. As a consequence, some anthropological gerontologists appear to feel less at home within anthropology at precisely the time when they were gaining a positive reception within gerontology. A loosening of ties to general anthropology, a reluctance to risk the newer crossdisciplinary connections, and a growing subspecialization and in-group affiliation may all contribute to what we believe to be a reluctance to become involved in the challenging but dynamic state of theory within anthropology. Substituting for this involvement is a pattern within anthropological gerontology of developing internally derived theories, e.g., modernization, and then testing these relatively narrow theories. Instead of examining the merits or demerits of macrotheories like structural Marxism or practice, anthropological gerontologists debate, modify, or dismiss the more narrow and specialized theories. In the short term, there are likely to be benefits from this approach, but in the long term this will dilute what anthropologists can offer as they become indistinguishable from their colleagues in gerontology.

REFERENCE

Almagor, U. (1978). The ethos of equality among Dassanetch age peers. In P.T.W. Baxter and U. Almagor (Eds.), *Age, Generation and Time,* pp. 69–94. New York: St. Martin's Press.

Amoss, P. T. (1981). Coast Salish elders. In P. T. Amoss and S. Harrell (Eds.), *Other Ways of Growing Old,* pp. 227–38. Stanford, Calif.: Stanford University Press.

Amoss, P. T., and Harrell, S. (Eds.) (1981). *Other Ways of Growing Old*. Stanford, Calif.: Stanford University Press.

Arnhoff, F. N., Leon, H. V., and Lorge, I. (1964). Cross-cultural acceptance of stereotypes toward aging. *Journal of Social Psychology, 63*, 41–58.

Arth, M. (1972). Aging: A cross-cultural perspective. In D. Kent, R. Kastenbaum, and S. Sherwood (Eds.), *Research Planning and Action for the Elderly*, pp. 352–64. New York: Behavioral Science Publishing.

Beattie, W. M. (1964). The place of older people in different societies. In P. Hanson (Ed.), *Age with a Future: Proceedings of the Sixth International Congress of Gerontology*. Philadelphia: F. A. Davis.

Beaubier, J. (1976). *High Life Expectancy on the Island of Paros, Greece*. New York: Philosophical Library.

Becker, G. (1983). *Growing Old in Silence: Deaf People in Old Age*. Berkeley and Los Angeles: University of California Press.

Benet, S. (1974). *Abkhasians: The Long-Lived People of the Caucausus*. New York: Holt, Rinehart and Winston.

Bengtson, V. L. et al. (1975). Modernization, modernity, and perceptions of aging: A cross-cultural study. *Journal of Gerontology, 30* (6), 688–95.

Bernardi, B. (1985). *Age Class Systems: Social Institutions and Policies Based on Age*. Cambridge: Cambridge University Press.

Biesele, M., and Howell, N. (1981). The old people give you life. In P. T. Amoss and S. Harrell (Eds.), *Other Ways of Growing Old*, pp. 77–92. Stanford, Calif.: Stanford University Press.

Bloch, M. (1974). The long term and the short term: The economic and political significance of the morality of kinship. In J. Goody (Ed.), *The Character of Kinship*. Cambridge: Cambridge University Press.

Bourdieu, P. (1978 [1972]). *Outline of a Theory of Practice*. Translated by R. Nice. Cambridge: Cambridge University Press.

Brown, J. K. (1981). Cross-cultural perspectives on the female life cycle. In R. H. Munroe, R. L. Munroe, and B. B. Whiting (Eds.), *Handbook of Cross-Cultural Human Development*. New York: Garland.

Brown, J. K. (1982). Cross-cultural perspectives on middle-aged women. *Current Anthropology, 23* (2), 143–56.

Clark, M. (1967). The anthropology of aging: A new area for studies of culture and personality. *The Gerontologist, 7*, 55–65.

Clark, M. (1973). Contributions of cultural anthropology to the study of the aged. In L. Nader and T. Maretski (Eds.), *Cultural Illness and Health*. Washington, D.C.: American Anthropological Association.

Clark, M., and Anderson, B. (1967). *Culture and Aging: An Anthropological Study of Older Americans*. Springfield, Ill.: Charles C. Thomas.

Clark, M., Kaufman, S., and Pierce, R. C. (1976). Explorations of acculturation: Toward a model of ethnic identity. *Human Organization, 35* (3), 231–37.

Cohen, C. I., and Sokolovsky, J. (1980). Social engagement versus isolation: The case of the aged in SRO hotels. *The Gerontologist, 20* (1), 36–44.

Colson, E., and Scudder, T. (1981). Old age in the Guembe District, Zambia. In P. T. Amoss and S. Harrell (Eds.), *Other Ways of Growing Old*, pp. 125–54. Stanford, Calif.: Stanford University Press.

Cool, L. E. (1980). Ethnic identity: A source of community esteem for the elderly. *Anthropological Quarterly,* 54, 179–89.

Cool, L. E. and McCabe, J. (1983). The scheming hag and the dear old thing: The anthropology of aging women. In J. Sokolovsky (Ed.), *Growing Old in Different Cultures,* pp. 56–68. Belmont, Calif.: Wadsworth.

Cowgill, D. O. (1974). Aging and modernization: A revision of the theory. In J. Gubrium (Ed.), *Communities and Environmental Policy,* pp. 123–46. Springfield, Ill.: Charles C. Thomas.

Cowgill, D. O., and Holmes, L. (1972). *Aging and Modernization.* New York: Appleton-Century-Crofts.

Cuellar, J. (1978). El senior citizens center. In B. Myerhoff and A. Simic (Eds.), *Aging: Life's Career.* Beverly Hills, Calif.: Sage.

Davis, D. (1975). *The Centenarians of the Andes.* Garden City, N.Y.: Anchor Press.

Delaney, B. (1981). Uncle Sam insane? Pride, humor and clique formation in a northern Thai home for the elderly. *International Journal of Aging and Human Development,* 13, 137–50.

deYoung, J. (1958). *Village Life in Modern Thailand.* Berkeley and Los Angeles: University of California Press.

Dolhinow, P. (1984). The primates: Age, behavior and evolution. In D. Kertzer and J. Keith (Eds.), *Age and Anthropological Theory,* pp. 65–81. Ithaca, N.Y.: Cornell University Press.

Dowd, J. J. (1980). *Stratification among the Aged.* Monterey, Calif.: Brooks/Cole.

Eckert, J. K. (1980). *The Unseen Elderly.* San Diego: The Campanile Press.

Eisenstadt, S. N. (1956). *From Generation to Generation.* New York: Free Press.

Featherman, D. (1981). *The Life Span Perspective in Social Science Research.* New York: Social Science Research Council.

Featherman, D. L., and Petersen, T. (1986). Markers of aging. *Research on Aging,* 8 (3), 339–65.

Finley, G. E. (1982). Modernization and aging. In T. Field et al. (Eds.), *Review of Human Development.* New York: Wiley Interscience.

Foner, A., and Kertzer, D. (1978). Transitions over the life course: Lessons from age-set societies. *American Journal of Sociology,* 83 (5), 1081–1104.

Foner, N. (1984a). Age and social change. In D. I. Kertzer and J. Keith (Eds.), *Age and Anthropological Theory,* pp. 195–219. Ithaca, N.Y.: Cornell University Press.

Foner, N. (1984b). *Ages in Conflict: A Cross-Cultural Perspective on Inequality between Old and Young.* New York: Columbia University Press.

Fortes, M. (1984). Age, generation and social structure. In D. I. Kertzer and J. Keith (Eds.), *Age and Anthropological Theory,* pp. 99–122. Ithaca, N.Y.: Cornell University Press.

Francis, D. G. (1984). *Will You Still Need Me, Will You Still Feed Me, When I'm 84?* Bloomington: Indiana University Press.

Friedman, J. (1974). Marxism, structuralism, and vulgar materialism. *Man,* 9 (3), 444–69.

Friedman, J. (1975). Tribes, states and transformations. In M. Bloch (Ed.), *Marxist Analyses and Social Anthropology.* New York: John Wiley and Sons.

Fries, J. F., and Crapo, L. M. (1981). *Vitality and Aging.* San Francisco: Freeman.

Fry, C. L. (1976). The ages of adulthood: A question of numbers. *Journal of Gerontology,* 31, 170–77.

Fry, C. L. (1981). *Dimensions: Aging, Culture and Health.* New York: Praeger.

Fry, C. L. (1985). Culture, behavior and aging in the comparative perspective. In J. Birren and K. Schaie (Eds.), *Handbook of the Psychology of Aging.* New York: Van Nostrand Reinhold.

Fry, C. L. (1988). Theories of age and culture. In J. E. Birren and V. L. Bengtson (Eds.), *Emergent Theories of Aging: Psychological and Social Perspectives on Time, Self, and Society,* pp. 1–54. New York: Springer Publishing.

Fry, C. L., and Keith, J. (1982). The life course as a cultural unit. In M. W. Riley, R. Ables, and M. Teitelbaum (Eds.), *Aging from Birth to Death: Sociotemporal Perspectives,* pp. 51–70. Boulder, Colo.: Westview Press.

Fry, C. L., and Keith, J. (1986). *New Methods for Old Age Research: Strategies for Studying Diversity.* South Hadley, Mass.: Bergin and Garvey.

Geertz, C. (1973). *The Interpretation of Cultures.* New York: Basic Books.

Geertz, C. (1975). On the nature of anthropological understanding. *The American Scientist,* 63 (1), 47–53.

Geertz, C. (1980). Blurred genres: The refiguration of social thought. *The American Scholar,* 49 (2), 165–79.

Glascock, A. P. (1982). Decrepitude and death-hastening: The nature of old age in third world societies. *Studies in Third World Societies,* 22, 43–67.

Glascock, A. P. (1986). Resource control among older males in southern Somalia. *Journal of Cross-Cultural Gerontology,* 1 (1), 51–73.

Glascock, A. P. (in press). The myth of the golden isle: Old age in pre-industrial societies. *Selected Papers Volume of the Eighth International Congress of Cross-Cultural Psychology.*

Goldstein, M. C., and Beall, C. M. (1981). Modernization and aging in the third and fourth world: Views from the rural Hinterland in Nepal. *Human Organization,* 40 (1), 48–55.

Goody, J. (1976). Aging in non-industrial societies. In R. H. Binstock and E. Shanas (Eds.), *Handbook of Aging and the Social Sciences,* pp. 117–29. New York: Van Nostrand Reinhold.

Guemple, L. (1969). Human resource management: The dilemma of the aging Eskimo. *Sociological Symposium,* 2, 59–74.

Guemple, L. (1983). Growing old in the Inuit society. In J. Sokolovsky (Ed.), *Growing Old in Different Societies.* Belmont, Calif.: Wadsworth.

Gutmann, D. (1974). Alternatives to disengagement: The old men of the highland Druze. In R. LeVine (Ed.), *Culture and Personality: Contemporary Readings,* pp. 232–45. Chicago: Aldine.

Gutmann, D. (1977). The cross-cultural perspective: Notes toward a comparative psychology of aging. In J. E. Birren and K. W. Schaie (Eds.), *Handbook of the Psychology of Aging,* pp. 302–26. New York: Van Nostrand Reinhold.

Hamer, J. H. (1972). Aging in gerontocratic society. The Sidamo of southwest Ethiopia. In D. O. Cowgill and L. D. Holmes (Eds.), *Aging and Modernization,* pp. 15–30. New York: Appleton-Century-Crofts.

Harlan, W. (1964). Social status of the aged in three Indian villages. *Vita Humana,* 7, 239–52.

Harrell, S. (1981). Growing old in rural Taiwan. In P. T. Amoss and S. Harrell (Eds.),

Other Ways of Growing Old, pp. 193–210. Stanford, Calif.: Stanford University Press.

Harris, M. (1969). The cultural ecology of India's sacred cattle. *Current Anthropology*, 7, 51–59.

Hendricks, J. (1982). The elderly in society: Beyond modernization. *Social Science History*, 4 (3), 321–45.

Holmes, L. D. (1976). Trends in anthropological gerontology: From Simmons to the seventies. *International Journal of Aging and Human Development*, 7, 211–20.

Holmes, L. D. (1983). *Other Cultures, Elder Years*. Minneapolis: Burgess Publishing.

Hornum, B. (1983). The elderly in British new towns: New roles, new networks. In J. Sokolovsky (Ed.), *Growing Old in Different Cultures*, pp. 211–24. Belmont, Calif.: Wadsworth.

Hrdy, S. B. (1981). Nepotists and altruists: The behavior of old females among Macaques and Langur monkeys. In P. T. Amoss and S. Harrell (Eds.), *Other Ways of Growing Old*, pp. 59–76. Stanford, Calif.: Stanford University Press.

Ikels, C. (1980). The coming of age in Chinese society: Traditional patterns and contemporary Hong Kong. In C. L. Fry (Ed.), *Aging in Culture and Society: Comparative Perspectives and Strategies*, pp. 80–100. New York: Praeger.

Jacobs, J. (1984). *Fun City: An Ethnographic Study of a Retirement Community*. New York: Holt, Rinehart and Winston.

Johnson, C. L. (1983). Interdependence and aging in Italian families. In J. Sokolovsky (Ed.), *Growing Old in Different Cultures*, pp. 92–103. Belmont, Calif.: Wadsworth.

Just, P. (1980). Time and leisure in the elaboration of culture. *Journal of Anthropological Research*, 36, 87–104.

Kapferer, B. (Ed.) (1976). *Transaction and Meaning: Directions in the Anthropology of Exchange and Human Behavior*. Philadelphia: ISHI Publications.

Katz, S. (1978). Anthropological perspectives on aging. *Annals*, 438, 1–20.

Kayser-Jones, J. S. (1981). *Old, Alone and Neglected: Care of the Aged in Scotland and the United States*. Berkeley: University of California Press.

Keith, J. (1979). The ethnography of old age. *Anthropological Quarterly*, 52, 1–69.

Keith, J. (1980). The best is yet to be: Toward an anthropology of age. *Annual Review of Anthropology*, 9, 339–64.

Keith, J. (1981). The back to anthropology movement in gerontology. In C. L. Fry (Ed.), *Dimensions: Aging, Culture, and Health: Comparative Perspectives and Strategies*, pp. 285–93. Brooklyn: J. F. Bergin Inc.

Keith, J. (1982). *Old People as People: Social and Cultural Influences on Aging and Old Age*. Boston: Little, Brown and Co.

Keith, J. (1985). Age in anthropological research. In R. Binstock and E. Shanas (Eds.), *Handbook of Aging and the Social Sciences*, pp. 231–63. New York: Van Nostrand Reinhold.

Kertzer, D. I. (1978). Theoretical developments in the study of age-group systems. *American Ethnologist*, 5, 368–74.

Kertzer, D. I., and Keith, J. (Eds.) (1984). *Age and Anthropological Theory*. Ithaca, N.Y.: Cornell University Press.

Kertzer, D. I., and Madison, O. B. B. (1981). Women's age-set systems in Africa: The Latuka of southern Sudan. In C. L. Fry (Ed.), *Dimensions: Aging, Culture and Health*, pp. 109–30. New York: Praeger.

Kiefer, C. W. (1971). Notes on anthropology and the minority elderly. *The Gerontologist,* Spring, pt. 2, 94–98.

LaFontaine, J. S. (1978). Introduction. In J. S. LaFontaine (Ed.), *Sex and Age as Principles of Social Differentiation,* pp. 1–20. New York: Academic Press.

Laslett, P. (1985). Societal development and aging. In R. Binstock and E. Shanas (Eds.), *Handbook of Aging and the Social Sciences.* 2d ed., pp. 199–230. New York: Van Nostrand Reinhold.

Lee, G. R., and Kezis, M. (1981). Societal literacy and the aged. *International Journal of Aging and Human Development,* 12, 221–34.

Lee, R. (1969). Kung bushmen subsistence: An input-output analysis. In A. Vayda (Ed.), *Environment and Cultural Behavior,* pp. 47–79. Garden City, N.Y.: The Natural History Press.

LeVine, R. (1978). Adulthood and aging in cross-cultural perspective. *Items,* 31 (12), 1–5.

Levi-Strauss, C. (1963). *Structural Anthropology.* Translated by C. Jacobson and B. G. Schoepf. New York: Basic Books.

Levi-Strauss, C. (1969). *The Elementary Structures of Kinship.* Translated by J. H. Bell and J. R. Von Sturmer and edited by R. Needham. Boston: Beacon Press.

Maxwell, R., and Silverman, P. (1970). Information and esteem: Cultural considerations in the treatment of the aged. *International Journal of Aging and Human Development,* 1, 361–92.

Maxwell, R., Silverman, P., and Maxwell, E. (1982). The motive for gerontologists. *Studies in Third World Societies,* 22, 67–84.

Maybury-Lewis, D. (1984). Age and kinship: A structural view. In D. I. Kertzer and J. Keith (Eds.), *Age and Anthropological Theory.* Ithaca, N.Y.: Cornell University Press.

Myerhoff, B. (1979). *Number Our Days.* New York: Dutton.

Myerhoff, B. (1984). Rites and signs of ripening: The intertwining of ritual, time and growing older. In D. I. Kertzer and J. Keith (Eds.), *Age and Anthropological Theory,* pp. 305–30. Ithaca, N.Y.: Cornell University Press.

Myerhoff, B., and Simic, A. (1978). *Life's Career—Aging: Cultural Variation in Growing Old.* Beverly Hills, Calif.: Sage.

Myers, G. C. (1985). Aging and worldwide population change. In R. H. Binstock and E. Shanas (Eds.), *Handbook of Aging and the Social Sciences.* 2d ed., pp. 173–98. New York: Van Nostrand Reinhold.

Needham, R. (1974). Age, category and descent. In R. Needham (Ed.), *Remarks and Inventions.* London: Tavistock.

Nydegger, C. N. (1981). On being caught in time. *Human Development,* 24, 1–12.

Nydegger, C. N. (1983). Family ties of the aged in cross-cultural perspective. *The Gerontologist,* 23 (1), 26–32.

Ortner, S. B. (1984). Theory in anthropology since the sixties. *Comparative Studies in Society and History,* 26 (1): 126–66.

Palmore, E. B. (1983). Cross-cultural research. *Research on Aging,* 5 (1), 45–57.

Palmore, E. B., and Manton, K. (1974). Modernization and status of the aged. *Journal of Gerontology,* 29, 205–10.

Piddocke, S. (1965). The potlatch system of the Southern Kwakiutl: A new perspective. *Southwest Journal of Anthropology,* 21, 244–64.

Plath, D. W. (1972). Japan: The after years. In D. O. Cowgill and L. Holmes (Eds.), *Aging and Modernization*, pp. 133–50. New York: Appleton-Century-Crofts.

Press, I., and McKool, M., Jr. (1972). Social structure and status of the aged: Toward some valid cross-cultural generalizations. *Aging and Human Development, 3*, 297–306.

Radcliffe-Brown, A. R. (1952). *Structure and Function in Primitive Society*. Glencoe, Ill.: The Free Press.

Rappaport, R. (1967). Ritual regulation among a New Guinea people. *Ethnology, 6*, 17–30.

Ritter, M. L. (1980). The conditions favoring age set organization. *Journal of Anthropological Research, 3*, 687–704.

Ross, J. (1977). *Old People, New Lives: Community Creation in a Retirement Residence*. Chicago: University of Chicago Press.

Sahlins, M., and Service, E. R. (Eds.) (1960). *Evolution and Culture*. Ann Arbor: University of Michigan Press.

Schepler-Hughs, N. (1983). Deposed kings: The demise of the rural Irish gerontocracy. In J. Sokolovsky (Ed.), *Growing Old in Different Cultures*, pp. 131–46. Belmont, Calif.: Wadsworth.

Schneider, J. (1978). Peacocks and penguins: The political economy of European cloth and colors. *American Ethnologist, 5* (3), 413–47.

Schneider, J., and Schneider, P. (1976). *Culture and Political Economy in Western Sociology*. New York: Academic Press.

Sheehan, T. (1976). Senior esteem as a factor in socioeconomic complexity. *The Gerontologist, 5*, 2–23.

Silverman, P., and Maxwell, R. J. (1978). How do I respect thee? Let me count the ways: Deference towards elderly men and women. *Behavioral Science Research, 13*, 91–108.

Simmons, L. (1945). *The Role of the Aged in Primitive Society*. New Haven: Yale University Press.

Simmons, L. (1960). Aging in pre-industrial societies. In C. Tibbitts (Ed.), *Handbook of Social Gerontology*, pp. 62–90. Chicago: University of Chicago Press.

Sokolovsky, J. (1981). Being old in the inner city: Support systems of the S.R.O. aged. In C. L. Fry (Ed.), *Dimensions: Aging, Culture and Health*. New York: Praeger.

Sokolovsky, J. (1982). Aging and the aged in the third world: Part I. *Studies in Third World Societies, 22*, 1–21.

Sokolovsky, J. (1983). *Growing Old in Different Societies*. Belmont, Calif.: Wadsworth.

Spencer, P. (1965). *The Samburu: A Study of Gerontocracy in a Nomadic Tribe*. London: Routledge and Kegan Paul.

Spencer, P. (1975). Opposing streams and the gerontocratic ladder: Two models of age organization in east Africa. *Man, 11*, 153–75.

Stearns, P. (1979). The evolution of traditional culture toward aging. In J. Hendricks and C. Hendricks (Eds.), *Dimensions of Aging*. Cambridge, Mass.: Winthrop.

Steward, J. H. (1953). Evolution and process. In A. L. Kroeber (Ed.), *Anthropology Today*. Chicago: University of Chicago Press.

Steward, J. H. (1955). *Theory of Culture Change*. Urbana: University of Illinois Press.

Streib, G. F. (1972). Old age in Ireland: Demographic and sociological aspects. In D. O. Cowgill and L. Holmes (Eds.), *Aging and Modernization*, pp. 167–81. New York: Appleton-Century-Crofts.

Townsend, P. (1964). The place of older people in different societies. In P. Hanson (Ed.), *Proceedings of the Sixth International Congress of Gerontology, Copenhagen, 1963*. Philadelphia: F. A. Davis.

Turner, V. (1967). *The Forest of Symbols*. Ithaca, N.Y.: Cornell University Press.

Turner, V. (1969). *The Ritual Process*. Chicago: Aldine.

Turton, D. (1978). Territorial organization and age among the Mursi. In P.T.W. Baxter and U. Almagor (Eds.), *Age, Generation and Time*, pp. 95–130. New York: St. Martin's Press.

Van Arsdale, P. W. (1981). Disintegration of the ritual support network among aged Asmat hunter-gatherers of New Guinea. In C. L. Fry (Ed.), *Dimensions: Aging, Culture and Health*, pp. 33–46. New York: Praeger.

Vatuk, S. (1980). Withdrawal and disengagement as a cultural response to aging in India. In C. L. Fry (Ed.), *Aging in Culture and Society: Comparative Perspectives and Strategies*. New York: Praeger.

Vesperi, M. D. (1986). *City of Green Benches: Growing Old in a New Downtown*. Ithaca, N.Y.: Cornell University Press.

Washburn, S. L. (1981). Longevity in primates. In J. L. McGaugh and S. B. Kiesler (Eds.), *Aging: Biology and Behavior*. New York: Academic Press.

Werner, D. (1981). Gerontocracy among the Mekranoti of central Brazil. *Anthropological Quarterly*, 54, 15–27.

White, L. A. (1943). Energy and the evolution of culture. *The American Anthropologist*, 45 (3), 335–56.

White, L. A. (1959). *The Evolution of Culture*. New York: McGraw-Hill.

Whiting, J.M.W. (1981). Aging and becoming an elder: A cross-cultural comparison. In R. W. Fogel (Ed.), *Aging: Stability and Change in the Family*. New York: Academic Press.

Wilson, M. (1951). *Good Company: Study of Nyakyusa Age Villages*. London: Oxford University Press.

Part II
THE PRACTICING DISCIPLINES

6. THE RELATIONSHIP OF GERIATRICS AND GERONTOLOGY: ON FORGING LINKS BETWEEN CURING AND CARING

Evan Calkins and Jurgis Karuza

Geriatrics and gerontology—the two terms, often interchangeable and imprecisely used, refer to two distinct professional and academic movements in the field of aging. Geriatrics is the branch of medicine concerned with the health of elderly persons, including the clinical, preventive, and social psychological aspects of illness and old age. Gerontology refers to the scientific study of aging as a biological and social phenomenon (Association of American Medical Colleges, 1983; Beck and Vivells, 1984; Birren and Clayton, 1975; Nascher, 1914; National Academy of Sciences, 1978).

Obviously, the two fields are, and must be, closely intertwined. This has not always been the case, however, especially in the United States. The lack of a constructive, informal, and mutually supportive interrelationship between geriatrics and gerontology, specifically its psychological and social aspects, represents one of the most important challenges to those concerned with the elderly— a challenge that requires a significant response if the needs of the elderly population, present and future, are to be met.

Any attempt to review, simultaneously, the historical development of two fields as distinct as geriatrics and gerontology is hazardous at best. Nevertheless, it is even more hazardous to attempt to understand the present and anticipate the future without a genuine effort to understand the past. In this spirit, it may be helpful to offer a few perspectives that may help students or practitioners in one field understand the other.

We start by reviewing some of the changes that have taken place within medicine and some of the reasons why clinical medicine in the United States is having difficulty in coping with the needs of the elderly. Second, we shift attention to gerontology and explore some of the reasons why social sciences' research and theory have not contributed to geriatric practice as fully as it could have. Finally, we consider some of the problems that emerge as physicians and gerontologists begin to work together and propose some suggestions for the future to facilitate the needed interdisciplinary linkages between geriatrics and gerontology.

MEDICAL CURE: A HISTORICAL PERSPECTIVE

It is paradoxical that two of the developments that have had a most profound and generally favorable influence on the quality of American medical care are developments that, at least in some ways, have proven detrimental to the development of a system of effective, comprehensive care for the elderly—i.e., good quality geriatrics. The first is the increasingly intense interrelationship between American medicine and the basic biomedical sciences and the second is the issue of "free choice of the physician" and, with it, the fee-for-service aspect of medical care.

Biomedical Basis of Clinical Medicine

The close association of clinical medicine and the biomedical sciences probably dates from the famous Flexner Report (1910). Based on an analysis of the then-current state of academic medicine in this country, the report recommended a number of changes in this educational system, including the establishment of strong basic science departments as integral components of a medical school and inclusion of education in the basic biomedical sciences as an essential ingredient in the education of all physicians. This wedding of the clinical and basic biomedical sciences established the pattern of academic medicine in the United States for decades to come. The identification of the white laboratory coat, as the proper garb of hospital-based physicians, is but one indication of the extent to which laboratory medicine became recognized as the proper base or style for institution-based physicians.

The tremendous advances in the biochemical and clinical sciences that have evolved from this association have enabled physicians to cure many acute conditions that they, in the past, were content to palliate. Medicine emerged, increasingly, as a "high tech" specialty (Starr, 1982). Given the robustness of biologically based interventions in acute cases, the downplaying of a social science perspective did not detract from the overall effectiveness of acute care medicine. Simultaneously, from the perspective of medical education, the tradition of forty years ago that physicians should be well-rounded people first and professionals second has been replaced by a model in which the ideal medical student excels in science and mathematics, with little emphasis placed on interpersonal skills and a background in the humanities. Throughout medical school, the major emphasis is focused on technological aspects, with little attention being given to the social sciences, to say nothing of management skills.

Understanding chronic conditions, however, especially in the elderly, requires a much broader focus, which includes consideration of psychological and social, as well as physiological, changes in the host organism. Responsiveness to these psychological and social aspects of individuals becomes important, not only in the sense of contributing to the quality of the interpersonal relationship between professional and patient, but also in providing better assessment criteria and quality of care indices. Individual characteristics of patients, such as motivation, functional level, and social support network, become additional resources for primary care clinicians as they work with patients and their families to develop primary prevention programs or interventions aimed at compensating for functional limits (Brickman et al., 1982).

Correspondingly, development of effective programs of care for the elderly requires not only the presence of physicians who are trained in and sensitive to psychosocial as well as biomedical issues, but also the development of a new style of care, one that employs an interdisciplinary approach. Physicians are increasingly required to work as members of a team along with other health and allied health specialists such as nurses, physical therapists, social workers, and psychologists in assessing the patient and orchestrating a treatment plan. It is interesting that the white coat has become such a symbol, not only of the scientific prowess of the physician but also of his or her authority and status, that some modern mental institutions, desirous of establishing effective patterns of team care, have forbidden its use.

Fee-for-Service and Freedom of Choice

A second dimension of American medicine that, we suggest, has had a profound influence on the course of geriatrics in this country and on the relationship of geriatrics and gerontology is the fee-for-service tradition of medicine and the closely related principle of free choice of a physician. The privilege of choosing the person to whom one trusts one's medical care and possibly one's life is as logical and American as apple pie. Having chosen the physician, to recognize the relationship by direct payment of his or her bill provides an important confirmation of this trust and would, logically, be thought to contribute significantly to the patient's confidence in the physician and compliance with his or her instructions. This pattern has emerged for decades as one of the fundamental principles of medicine in the United States, staunchly defended by the American Medical Association.

As the practice of medicine moves into an era of comprehensive, prevention-oriented care, as required by the elderly, problems emerge with this arrangement. In an interdisciplinary method of care, does one also have free choice of a nurse practitioner? or a social worker? or a dietician or occupational therapist? If so, what assurance does one receive that these people, accustomed to operating independently, will be able to work together effectively as a team? What happens to the fee-for-service concept as the health care system moves to prepaid medical care, with increasing reliance toward the corporate health care system as the source of services and third-party reimbursement as the source of payment? (Freedman, 1985.)

An additional problem for many physicians, patients, and the health care system as a whole is the wide discrepancy between the income available to the procedure-oriented subspecialist, such as the cardiologist or neurologist, with their complex technical procedures for which they receive handsome remuneration, as opposed to the much more limited remuneration associated with comprehensive primary care. It is inescapable that the fee-for-service tradition has led to a tendency of physicians to overuse these expensive procedures and to place less emphasis on the "hands on" skills of history taking and physical examination. The result is a further depersonalization of the patterns of care and an almost certain increase in the cost of medical care.

In addition to providing serious barriers to the development of effective programs of interdisciplinary team care, the fee-for-service tradition has additional adverse effects both on the economic status of the allied health professionals and on the extent to which these professionals can employ their skills for the benefit of their patients. This has been accomplished by fostering the development of regulations that limit practice privileges for clinical professions in the health and health-related disciplines. As a result, physicians and other health and health-related professionals become increasingly isolated from each other. Frequently heard cries of unfair competition among physicians, nurses, social workers, and psychologists and disciplinary based jealousies and rivalries make it difficult to forge interdisciplinary efforts (Uyeda and Moldawsky, 1986).

An especially damaging by-product of this is that many health professionals from a number of disciplines decline to treat the elderly. For example, only 2 to 3 percent of psychologists currently practice with the elderly (Uyeda and Moldawsky, 1986). Not only are psychology resources underused, but the lack of expertise and commitment to geropsychology makes it difficult to recruit and train students within psychology who could work in geriatric settings and stifles applied geriatric research efforts.

In summary, the last fifty years have seen American medicine, especially "technical medicine," evolve to a position of world preeminence. Paradoxically, several of the characteristics of the field that have played an important role in this achievement have created major problems as this health care system begins to address the needs of the elderly. These characteristics also create special problems in the interface between geriatrics and gerontology, problems that need to be addressed if the elderly are to receive the type of care they need.

INSULARITY OF GERONTOLOGY

A good portion of the blame for the isolation of geriatrics and gerontology from each other lies also with the approach of gerontologists, in particular those in the social sciences. While it is true that the gerontology literature has grown logarithmically (Birren and Clayton, 1975), several critics have pointed out that this has created a confusing surfeit that makes access to relevant scholarly works difficult (Riegel, 1973). Even with lip service paid to the multidisciplinary nature of gerontology, many of the articles tend to be very specialized, not only within disciplinary units but within disciplinary subspecialties, with little interdisciplinary cooperation or crossfertilization. Given the pressures of academe, many of these articles appear to be more important for the competitive success of gerontology scholars within their discipline, rather than for the growth or betterment of the human condition.

Especially dangerous is the "instant gerontologist" phenomenon (Seltzer, 1979)—faculty members who jump on the gerontology bandwagon without a firm understanding of the dynamics of aging. Rather than appreciating the manifold complexity of the aging process, they often impose their narrow disciplinary perspective on the research or teaching issues at hand, much like a five-year-old playing with a hammer, turning the whole world into a nail. The result is stilted and limiting scholarship that frequently perpetuates stereotypic views of aging.

Often, gerontology researchers' assumptions about aging processes make it difficult to integrate the biological and the psychosocial antecedents and consequences of aging (see Karuza et al., 1986). Typically, research follows one of two distinct paths, which can be seen in many of the now "classic" debates in gerontology—for example, disengagement theory versus activity theory; myth versus reality of intellectual decline in old age; and the compression versus expansion of morbidity. One response has been to accept aging as a period of decline, driven by inevitable senescent processes, and to buy into a biological prepotency/biological predetermination logic. Since decline in late life is seen as normal with little compensation to be expected, little room is left for innovative treatment options. The second response has been to deny the prepotency of biological processes and the declines associated with old age and focus on psychosocial variables and the potentials of elderly to be active, wise, and autonomous, in order to maximize the likelihood of successfully dealing with functional deficits. This rosy view of old age flies in the face of the real biological, psychological, and social problems facing many elderly and the challenges confronting the practitioner. Neither approach is very helpful in linking research and practice. Furthermore, this trap makes crossdisciplinary dialogues difficult and perpetuates the insularity of much of gerontology research and teaching from practice issues.

The mutual interdependence between gerontology research and geriatric practice needs to be reaffirmed. As geriatrics adopts primary care approaches, research on cognitive processes, emotional functioning, and social dynamics can be useful in developing better assessment tools for geriatric practitioners. This research can also be the wellspring for innovative mental health therapies and interventions such as training programs that can help elderly patients compensate for functional losses or develop their potentials. In turn, issues surrounding the practice of geriatrics define the reality of aging today and in the future. Changes in prevalence of chronic conditions, changes in functional level, increased reliance on community-based care and supports, and emphasis on prevention are some examples. Gerontological research on topics such as plasticity in cognitive functioning, psychology of control, life satisfaction, and social supports should consider the implications of these changes. Potential future concerns such as rationing health care resources or the legal implications of "Do Not Resuscitate" orders in nursing homes raise new issues for research on attitudes, quality of life, social justice, and autonomy, just to name a few topics.

Another reason for the lack of effective bridges between geriatric practice and gerontology research in the social sciences has been the isolation of many gerontologists from the arenas of practice. Often this starts with the graduate training of many social science programs. For example, a survey by Division 20, Adult Development and Aging, of the American Psychological Association found that very few, if any, geropsychology training programs had a clinical community or community orientation and only 15 percent reported an interdisciplinary knowledge or training base (see Stenmark and Dunn, 1982). Even the work settings for the novice social scientist/allied health practitioner and for the fledgling physician are kept apart to a considerable degree—the geriatric social worker or psychologist intern with his or her secure place within a community-based agency or institution; the young physician-in-training seldom emerging outside the doors of the tertiary care hospital.

THE CURRENT STATUS OF INTERDISCIPLINARY AND INTERINSTITUTIONAL COLLABORATION

Geriatric medicine challenges many of the assumptions of the traditional biomedical, fee-for-service, tertiary care, disciplinary based medical approach.

The approach of geriatric medicine, as opposed to the traditional pattern of medicine, is illustrated in Table 6.1. In particular, the goals of geriatric medicine can be summarized as follows: (1) preservation of functional capacity and independence, along with preservation of life; (2) prevention of acute illnesses and accidents, and attention to chronic illness along with acute care; and (3) attention to psychological, social, and socioeconomic antecedents and consequences of illness (see Association of American Medical Colleges, 1983; Beck and Vivells, 1984; Cassel and Walsh, 1984; Calkins, 1985; Calkins, 1987; Calkins, Davis, and Ford, 1986; National Academy of Sciences, 1978).

Achievement of these goals requires the establishment of an entirely new framework of interrelationships in the medical and social sciences and between the medical faculty and community in which it resides.

Over the past ten years, stimulated by the formation of the National Institute on Aging, and several important national studies and reports (for example, Cane et al. [1981]; Committee on Leadership in Academic Geriatric Medicine [1987]; Steele et al. [1987]; and the United States Senate Sub-Committee on Long Term Care of the Special Committee on Aging [1975]), programs in geriatric medicine

Table 6.1

Traditional Medicine and Modern Geriatric Medicine

Traditional Medicine	Modern Geriatric Medicine
Physician dominated Academic activities based, primarily, in tertiary care hospital	Interdisciplinary approach Broadly based in clinics, offices, nursing homes, senior centers, and patients' homes
Oriented to in-patients Rarely involves care of patients in nursing home	Major emphasis--ambulatory and home care Regular responsibility for nursing home patients
Minimal relationship with community agencies (agencies on aging, home care agencies, etc.)	Very close relationship with these agencies
Major emphasis on intermittent acute care; less emphasis on prevention	Major emphasis on prevention
Little emphasis on rehabilitation	Major emphasis on rehabilitation, to maintain function and independence
Primarily concerned with "medical issues"--i.e., applied biology	Equal concern for psychosocial issues
Heavy reliance on subspecialists' procedures	Major emphasis on comprehensive primary care, with specialists used for consultation only as needed

with the goals and characteristics described above have been developed in approximately one-third of this country's medical schools (Calkins, 1985; Robbins et al., 1982). The growth of the field has been carefully documented by Beck and his colleagues (1984). The gaps in the interrelationships between the social sciences and the health sciences (especially medicine), between medicine and the allied health professions (e.g., clinical psychologists, social workers, rehabilitation therapists), and between the health science campus and community agencies have begun to be addressed.

As the medical establishment and geriatric allied health professionals begin to work together, the relationship is not always smooth. In the academic setting, the very substantial increases in the level of financial support available for biomedical research in aging, as contrasted with the modest framework of funds available for research in the behavioral aspects, have led to understandable resentment. This may have been heightened with the decision of several universities to replace retiring heads of university gerontology centers and programs, previously focused on psychosocial issues, with biomedical scientists (see, for example, recent appointments at Duke, the University of Michigan, and the Andrus Center at the University of Southern California).

Clearly, if the strengths of gerontology and geriatric medicine are to be brought together at last, a substantial effort must be made by members of each group to appreciate their own strengths and modus operandi as well as those of the other, and to develop patterns that will be productive for all.

As a start, allied health professionals, academic gerontologists, community-based medical practitioners, and academic physicians need to learn a great deal more about the operating framework in which each group functions. For example, the relationship between clinical sites, on one hand, and academic programs, on the other, is different for medicine and the social sciences. While the administrative and decision-making personnel in the community sites usually have a background in the allied health professions or advanced social science degrees (such as in social work or psychology), the relationship between the community and the organized academic disciplines is usually, though not always, somewhat remote. Relatively few community-based administrators of Agencies on Aging or other service agencies serve as members of the adjunct faculty in academic departments in related disciplines. Relatively little crosscontact exists between the administrators' professional organizations and the more academic and disciplinary based professional associations.

In the health disciplines, the relationship between the community practitioner and the corresponding university organization varies markedly within each discipline. In nursing, there is, in most instances, a sharp division between the staff of hospitals, even in those institutions that are affiliated with the university in question, and the campus-based faculty. On the other hand, the relationship between the university medical faculty and the medical staff of the affiliated teaching hospital is so close as to be indistinguishable. In medical school faculties, the sense of uncertainty and paranoia, if it exists, tends to be on the part of the basic science faculty members, who may feel somewhat overwhelmed by the numbers and financial resources available to the hospital-based clinical faculty.

Paradoxically, almost without exception, the close relationship between academic medicine teaching faculty and practitioners (i.e., staff physicians) ends at the door of the university hospital. In the present tradition of American academic medicine, the boundaries of the academy have been sharply drawn so as to exclude, almost entirely, the range of activities taking place in private physicians' offices, community-based clinics, and patients' homes. The most notable exceptions to this dictum, Departments of Family Medicine, have, at least in New York State, been established through legislative action, often over strong protest from the academically based faculty.

If the relationships between the praxis and academics *within* the fields of health and social sciences are varied and complex, the relationships become more complex as one crosses disciplinary boundaries. Allied health professionals (at least some of whom harbor, for various reasons, deep-seated jealousy of physicians) resent the domineering habits of many physicians, their apparent lack of concern for psychosocial issues, and their disrespect for the bureaucracy that is emerging in community-based care. Administrators and care providers in community agencies are often deeply frustrated by the lack of cooperation and understanding and even the secretiveness of medical practitioners.

Conversely, members of the medical establishment usually feel distinctly uncomfortable in their relationship with community-based institutions that are devoted to social support and home care issues. The administrative structure is quite unfamiliar to them, and the science appears "soft." Physicians are puzzled as to why the dominant role they play within tertiary care hospitals is not reproduced in these community settings. The complex structure of the community-based services and support agencies appears totally bewildering. This gap in communication is rendered all the more deleterious when one recognizes the extent to which the precise words used in formulating the medical diagnosis serve as the path of entry into the community-based service system, since the eligibility for services, and for third-party payments, is often contingent on these medical assessments and diagnosis.

Additional factors, tending to isolate the social support and clinical systems, include the widely divergent levels of remuneration, reimbursement eligibility for the community-based services, and the varying levels of preparation required for entry into the various professions. A good number of social support and in-home support services are not currently covered by existing government-sponsored programs or third-party insurance. One current notorious example is Medicare's frequent denial of reimbursement for in-home services. In this era of the monetarization of health care, limited reimbursement is damning, not only because of limited funds but also because these services and the professionals who offer them are easily perceived as nonessential, unexciting, and second class. This is unfortunate, since these programs are the very bedrock for a coherent community-based primary care effort.

It is understandable, therefore, that efforts to develop close interrelationships between the social and clinical sciences have been marked by resentments, misunderstandings, and jealousies, rather than a spirit of effective cooperation. One is reminded of the complaint to the effect that "the medical model has failed."

CHALLENGE FOR THE FUTURE: DEVELOPMENT OF NEW ORGANIZATIONAL STRUCTURES

Recognition of the need to break down the boundaries between medicine, the allied health disciplines, and social sciences, as well as to begin to achieve effective linkages among these groups, began to emerge as national policy in the late 1970s. Two major national programs were developed—the Long Term Care Gerontology Centers, conceived and sponsored by the Administration on Aging, and the Geriatric Education Centers, initiated by the Bureau of Health

Professions. These two agencies, together with the Veterans Administration, the National Institute on Aging, and a number of private foundations, have identified a balanced commitment between the biomedical and social and psychological aspects of aging and care of the elderly as topics of major concern.

A description of each of these programs is beyond our scope in this chapter. Yet suffice it to say that most of these programs are characterized by several "core" ingredients. These include: (1) the assignment of relatively equal emphasis and decision-making importance to the allied health and health components, including medicine; (2) a matrix rather than hierarchical organizational structure; and (3) close interrelationships between community agencies and academic programs. This stands in contrast to the current trend of medical practice, with its emphasis on economic incentives and hierarchical structure.

If the reader follows our logic to this point, it will become apparent that, in our view, the future of geriatric practice and the study of aging requires the achievement of a new collaborative framework among health and allied health practitioners and the social sciences. Based on our selective historical review, we come away with the feeling that the time may be right for new approaches to organization.

Some generalizations may be pertinent here to help trace out a preliminary blueprint for future consideration. In our experiences (Feather et al., 1988; Karuza et al., 1988), we are beginning to find that an effective, close, and mutually supportive relationship between the medical and social sciences can be attained both in community sites and on campus. The probability of achieving these relationships is greatly enhanced by moving away from a marketplace logic to a "resource exchange" networking style (Sarason et al., 1977).

To bribe the participation of the other person simply by providing part of his or her salary, or supplemental income, does not work in the long run. Professionals, whether they be in the university or in the practice setting, are not motivated primarily by monetary goals. Instead, they are motivated by a desire to be effective in their roles and be productive and creative. Implicit in our argument is that the future of geriatrics depends on professionals transcending the current "yuppie" cultural ethos that uses monetary gain as the motivation and metric for success. The reliance on the carrot and stick of reimbursement mechanisms to achieve health policy goals, currently in vogue, serves in many ways to further reinforce the preoccupation with monetary issues among geriatricians and administrators.

It is important that geriatric professionals maintain a reasonable standard of living, but to define professional allegiance solely in terms of an extrinsic motivation to "make money" is counterproductive. With everyone asking "where's mine" or "what's it worth to me," an atmosphere of cooperation among colleagues and among the health and allied health disciplines is easily polluted. The resultant deterioration of crossdisciplinary and institutional linkages only serves to undermine the effectiveness of the primary care efforts. Ironically, in an era where health care policy decisions are sensitive to cost-effectiveness ratios, this trend can be deadly. Furthermore, the preoccupation with economic rewards can lead practitioners to become jaded or, as Jaqueline Leavitt, one of our physician colleagues puts it, to forget the "fun" in geriatrics—the joy of seeing patients retain independence, the satisfaction in working with other dedicated professionals. The long-term effect of becoming a "geriatric mercenary" on the quality of care and on one's own life satisfaction is an interesting question worth pursuing.

Our experiences suggest also that a close examination of the extraordinary commitment that modern American society has made to a hierarchical, disciplinary based professionalism is warranted. All too often, as currently carried out, quality is judged, not by outcome—the overall impact or effectiveness of the group as a whole—but by the extent to which each participating group or person possesses knowledge judged to be requisite within his or her field, meeting certain specific and individual standards. Whether a person's value should be measured, also, by his or her effect on fellow colleagues or impact on his or her home institution in helping it fulfill its mandate is a concept that is seldom assessed by inspectors or supervisors, be they from government or academic life. To break down disciplinary barriers between geriatrics and gerontology and between academe and practice requires such a recognition and valuing of interdisciplinary efforts.

The alternative is an organizational and administrative structure that is built on the mutual respect of colleagues, be they from the social sciences and allied health professions or the health sciences, or from the realms of community practice or academic life. These are people who work together by choice, not because of official mandate. One does not need to have administrative power, authority, or even official permission to achieve a relationship of this sort. Indeed, in our experience, the formal definition of structure, responsibility, and organizational interrelationships may be counterproductive to the success of the effort.

We are bold to suggest that entirely new organizational structures may, in time, emerge—structures that will bring together in new ways those who are concerned with care and those who devote their energies primarily to curing. In a recent visit, Reverend Robert Smith, chaplain to the staff of the State University of New York at Stony Brook Medical Center, pointed out that many aspects of modern, fragmented life are reminiscent of Europe in the fourth century. Then, with the dissolution of the Roman Empire, one saw the development of many new and transcending communities based on emergent ties. Some of these, such as nascent transnational trading communities, provided social bonds where there were few other arenas in which to grow. Others, such as the great monastic communities, provided an institutional continuity for nearly one thousand years. Today, those who seek to establish new relationships between social support systems and social science, between systems of health care and the medical sciences, may well be in the process of creating such "new communities" that will permit more idealistic and associational goals of this historic sort to evolve. For those of us who are well-ensconced within traditional professions, this is a

startling and novel idea. However, it provides a thought-provoking perspective
of how geriatrics and gerontology could and should interrelate.

REFERENCES

Association of American Medical Colleges (1983). *Proceedings of the Regional Institutes on Geriatrics and Medical Education.* Washington, D.C.: Association of American Medical Colleges.

Beck, J., and Vivells, S. (1984). The development of geriatrics in the United States. In C. K. Cassel and J. R. Walsh (Eds.), *Geriatric Medicine. Vol. II. Fundamentals of Geriatric Care.* New York: Springer-Verlag.

Birren, J. E., and Clayton, V. (1975). History of gerontology. In D. Woodruff and J. Birren (Eds.), *Aging.* New York: D. Van Nostrand.

Brickman, P.; Rabinowitz, V.; Karuza, J., Jr.; Coates, D.; Cohn, E.; and Kidder, L. (1982). Models of helping and coping. *American Psychologist,* 37, 368–84.

Calkins, E. (1985). Residency training in geriatric medicine—1984. *Bulletin New York Academy of Medicine,* 61 (1), 534–42.

Calkins, E. (1987). Geriatrics and the revolution in health care. *Journal of the American Geriatric Society,* 35, 696–99.

Calkins, E., Davis, P. I., and Ford, A. B. (Eds.) (1986). *Practice of Geriatrics.* Philadelphia: W. B. Saunders.

Cane, R. L. et al. (1981). *Geriatrics in the United States: Manpower Projections and Training Considerations.* Lexington, Mass.: D. C. Heath.

Cassel, C. K., and Walsh, J. R. (Eds.) (1984). *Geriatric Medicine. Vol. II. Fundamentals of Geriatric Care.* New York: Springer-Verlag.

Committee on Leadership in Academic Geriatric Medicine (1987). Report of institute on medicine: Academic geriatrics for the year 2000. *Journal of the American Geriatric Society,* 35, 773–91.

Feather, J.; Calkins, E.; Karuza, J., Jr.; and MacKellar, M. (1988). Interdisciplinary faculty training in geriatrics and gerontology: A non-clinical model. *Gerontology and Geriatric Education,* 8, 165–79.

Flexner, A. (1910). *Medical Education in the United States and Canada, Bulletin No. 4.* New York: Carnegie Foundation for the Advancement of Teaching.

Freedman, S. A. (1985). Megacorporate health care: A choice for the future. *New England Journal of Medicine,* 312 (9), 579–82.

Karuza, J., Jr.; Calkins, E.; Duffey, J.; and Feather, J. (1988). Networking in aging: A challenge, model, and evaluation. *Gerontologist,* 28, 147–55.

Karuza, J., Jr., Rabinowitz, V., and Zevon, M. A. (1986). Implications of control and responsibility on helping the aged. In M. Baltes and P. Baltes (Eds.), *The Psychology of Control and Aging.* Hillsdale, N.J.: Erlbaum.

Nascher, I. L. (1914). *Geriatrics: The Diseases of Old Age and Their Treatment.* Philadelphia: Blakiston's Son & Co.

National Academy of Sciences (1978). *Institute of Medicine: Report of a Study: Aging and Medical Education.* Washington, D.C.: National Academy of Sciences.

Riegel, K. F. (1973). On the history of psychological gerontology. In C. Eisdorfer and M. P. Lawton (Eds.), *The Psychology of Adult Development and Aging.* Washington, D.C.: American Psychological Association.

Robbins, A. S., Vivells, S., and Beck, J. (1982). A study of geriatric training programs in the United States. *Journal of Medical Education,* 57, 79–86.

Sarason, S. et al. (1977). *Human Services and Resource Networks.* San Francisco: Jossey-Bass.

Seltzer, M. M. (1979). Reflections on the phenomenon of the instant gerontologist. In H. Sterns et al. (Eds.), *Gerontology in Higher Education.* Belmont, Calif.: Wadsworth.

Starr, P. (1982). *The Social Transformation of American Medicine.* New York: Basic Books.

Steele, K. et al. (1987). Guidelines for fellowship training programs in geriatric medicine. *Journal of the American Geriatric Society,* 35, 792–95.

Stenmark, D. E., and Dunn, V. K. (1982). Issues related to the training of geropsychologists. In J. Santos and G. VandenBos (Eds.), *Psychology and the Older Adult: Challenges for Training in the 1980s.* Washington, D.C.: American Psychological Association.

United States Senate Sub-Committee on Long Term Care of the Special Committee on Aging (1975). *Nursing Home Care in the United States: Failure in Public Policy.* Washington, D.C.: U.S. Government Printing Office.

Uyeda, M. K., and Moldawsky, S. (1986). Prospective payment and psychological services: What difference does it make? Psychologists aren't in Medicare anyway! *American Psychologist,* 41, 60–63.

7. BACKGROUND TO COUNSELING THE ELDERLY: PERSPECTIVES FROM COUNSELING PSYCHOLOGY

Roselle Acerno Kalosieh and Joseph Pedoto

Over the last decade, the issue of counseling care for the elderly has come into sharper focus as a result of epidemiological studies examining the prevalence of psychological impairment in later life. A minimum of 10 percent of people over age sixty-five suffer some emotional or cognitive problem requiring professional assistance (U.S. DHEW, 1979). Other less conservative estimates for persons sixty-five and older residing in community settings range from 15 percent for the young-old to 25 percent for the oldest adults (Shanas and Maddox, 1985). Situational depression is the most common of psychiatric disorders affecting the elderly. Depression warranting intervention is estimated to affect 10 to 15 percent of the total geriatric population (Gurland and Cross, 1982), while an incidence as high as 60 percent is attributed to the institutionalized aged (Blazer, 1982).

Such disparate figures appear with great frequency in the gerontological psychology literature and give credence to the notion, shared by some researchers, that definitive and comprehensive research on psychiatric symptomatology in the aged has yet to be undertaken (LaRue, Dessonville, and Jarvik, 1985; Stenmark and Dunn, 1982). No doubt, much research on the emotional health of the elderly has been confounded due to a number of recurring methodological flaws. These include: small sample sizes, insensitive evaluation and analysis of research data, and inaccurate differential diagnosis of mental disorders (e.g., somatic and cognitive disturbances attendant to normal aging process interpreted as symptoms of depression). It is therefore not surprising that even the traditional belief that the elderly suffer a greater incidence of mental illness than other groups has been challenged by data from a recent NIMH study (1984). This study suggests that rates for specific mental disorders may actually be lower for the aged (Weissman et al., 1985).

UTILIZATION OF MENTAL HEALTH SERVICES

As opposed to the differences previously cited, there is virtually no disagreement regarding the elderly's extreme underutilization of specialty mental health services, whether public or private, in comparison with other groups (Goldstrom et al., 1987). Surveys of utilization of mental health centers, over the last twenty years, have remained remarkably consistent in reporting low usage (4 to 6 percent) of all services offered (Redick et al., 1973; Fleming et al., 1984). Recent data for office-based psychiatric consultation is similar in that only 4 percent of clientele are sixty-five and over (Schurman, Kramer, and Mitchell, 1985). The numerous possible explanations for disuse include: lack of access caused by immobility, inadequate transportation, financial restrictions, Medicare reimbursement policies, and the general attitudes of the elderly toward mental health treatment (Goldstrom et al., 1987). However, instead of colluding with a "blaming the victim" mentality, it is the authors' contention that the counseling profession must adopt a proactive rather than reactive posture toward the delivery of counseling services to the elderly.

HISTORY OF COUNSELING THE ELDERLY

The counseling profession, as a whole, has historically been slow to recognize and serve the needs of the elderly. Negative stereotypic beliefs concerning the efficacy of treatment for the aged can be traced back to Freud who suggested that near or about age fifty people lose the mental elasticity required to be reeducated through the therapeutic process (Freud, 1924). Over the years, this "static concept" of aging has been challenged by a number of theorists who conceive of aging as a "dynamic process" (Blum, 1977). For example, Maslow has discussed the lifelong process of self-actualization while Jung has labeled individuation as a developmental task of senescence (Jung, 1933; Maslow, 1954). It is arguable, however, that the greatest impact on the thinking of American psychologists regarding the elderly has been achieved by Erikson within the context of his eight-stage theory of ego development (Erikson, 1950). The Eriksonian model, which will be discussed in greater detail later, is an important progenitor of the life span/developmental approaches of numerous gerontological psychologists writing since the late fifties and early sixties (i.e., Neugarten and Kastenbaum among others). Despite progress, work in this area is far from complete. For example, Neugarten has suggested that few good developmental studies of the elderly have been undertaken. By the same token, in a more applied area, it has also been noted that relatively little training for counseling the elderly is available (Storandt, 1983). In a positive vein, Blum (1977) has offered at least one proposal for graduate curriculum development in psychology.

All in all, it is likely that significant misperception of the elderly still exists today in the counseling field. Blau and Berezin (1982) have pointed out that counselor values are merely a reflection of societal values concerning the aged.

As such, it is conceivable that many counselors may still feel that the elderly are poor candidates for therapy. The common equation of senescence with rigidity, organic dysfunction, and psychotic disorders, however, is not supported by recent evidence from the literature. Available statistics suggest that only 4 to 6 percent of those between age sixty-five and eighty-five suffer organic brain dysfunction (Hendricks and Hendricks, 1986) while only 5 to 10 percent of those sixty-five or older have diagnoses of moderate to severe mental disorders (Gurland and Cross, 1982).

DEVELOPMENTAL APPROACH TOWARD AGING

Whatever the reason for the predominant professional posture toward the elderly, it is nonetheless apparent that a significant number of nonorganic and nonpsychotic elderly individuals could benefit from counseling intervention. This group would include those aged individuals struggling with life crises. This decidedly developmental bent toward understanding the aging process in its entirety, including both normal and dysfunctional components, is a hallmark of counseling psychology. In particular, over the past twenty years, life span models have begun making inroads into applied areas of counseling in the form of psychoeducational interventions (Larsen, 1984). An important emphasis of most psychoeducational models is the maintenance of an adequate level of functioning. It is particularly pertinent to the elderly due to the fact that they face various normative life crises concurrent with diminishing resources in many areas. As Nancy Osgood has aptly reiterated: "Old age has been described as a season of losses—whether they be emotional, familial, physical, financial or otherwise" (Osgood and McIntosh, 1986). We will consider some of these losses in terms of expected life tasks and their concomitant psychological impact.

TASKS AND TRANSITIONS IN OLD AGE

What constitutes adequate functioning or adequate adjustment to old age? Life span and psychoeducational models have determined a series of later life transitions, each with its concomitant set of tasks as a yardstick to measure how well an individual is coping. It is important to mention at this point that each person's response to changes in later life evolves from his/her earlier life patterns. How the individual adjusts depends largely on the coping mechanisms employed during his/her lifetime and the flexibility of these mechanisms in the face of loss and new demands. Life patterns at one time functional may become dysfunctional with changing life cycle tasks (Howells, 1975).

These transition points will be explicated with the inherent tasks they pose for the aging adult.

1. *Launching*. The launching of the last child ushers in a new pattern of life and relationships in the second half of life (Deutscher, 1964). With children on their own, parents find they must focus on the marital dyad. For women, loss

in the maternal role function may cause adjustment problems, depending on the quality of the conjugal relationship and nature of the attachment to the child. Neugarten (1970) has noted that, contrary to popular opinion, most women adjust well to the "empty nest" transition. This stage and the "clean break" it involves are further complicated at this point in our culture by not only the departure of children from the home, but also through their frequent reentry through divorce and financial difficulties. The social and economic structure of present-day society keeps many parents on a "see-saw" in this regard. In families that are one child oriented, either through culture, biology, pathology, or other reasons, parents are never sure about how permanent this stage is. The "empty nest" may be a myth for many couples today, especially the poor. This, of course, complicates the establishment of a postparental marital relationship. Current research, however, supports the fact that after the satisfactory launching of children from the household, most couples experience increased marital satisfaction (Rollins and Feldman, 1970). Companionship, mutual caretaking, and sexual intimacy become highly valued as they once were in courtship and early marital life.

2. *Retirement.* Perhaps the most significant adjustment of later life is represented by retirement, especially since occupational success is the most prized goal in American culture (Williams, 1970). Retirement means more than the loss of a meaningful job role and income. Because of the status and power that our society gives to productivity, the loss of a job very often means loss of a sense of self-esteem and personal worth. Most women, even if they work outside the home, maintain role continuity as homemakers. Their task seems to be coping with their husbands' retirement (Heyman, 1970). This period may be further complicated by change of residence and the dislocation—if not disconnectedness with the social network—that this entails.

3. *Widowhood.* A chief concern of women is the prospect of widowhood (Neugarten and Weinstein, 1968). Women are four times as likely as men to be the survivor of marriage and more likely to be widowed at an earlier age. For men and women alike, the loss of a mate after a lifetime together presents a formidable adjustment. Financially, this time may be more difficult for the surviving woman if the man was the major breadwinner, but, socially, this is more difficult for men, who are usually linked to family and community through their wives. Given the longer life expectancy, we may well see more remarriage than in the past (Cleveland and Gianturco, 1976). Additionally, despite the social stigma, many older couples are cohabiting without marriage because of economic constraints.

4. *Illness and Death.* We have previously stated that old age is a time of multiple losses. Concomitant with losses in the economic, social, and psychological spheres is the loss of physical health. Impairment of physical and/or mental functioning, chronic pain, and progressively degenerating conditions are more prevalent in the old adult population than in any other group. This physical deterioration may be exacerbated by loneliness, depression, and hopelessness.

Unlike illnesses during prior phases of the life cycle, the maladies of old age are less likely to terminate in recovery. One must come to terms with his/her mortality. Denial of one's demise is difficult as one witnesses the death of friends and loved ones. Many who have spent years working with the elderly feel that older adults do not have a fear of death. Some elderly see it as the natural culmination to life; for others, it is a relief from the pain of illness. For many, religious and philosophical convictions can be of tremendous support in the face of death.

We have attempted to make the reader aware of some of the more significant life transitions of late life. Although most of the elderly will negotiate these transitions with a reasonable degree of success, others will not be successful. Next, we shall examine the reasons and remedies for late-age dysfunction in greater detail.

MALADAPTION IN OLD AGE

The foregoing discussion of losses routinely encountered by the elderly belies the popular conception of old age as a predominantly quiescent period that precedes death. Within the general context of diminishing personal resources endured by the aged, one may also recognize the potential for psychological dysfunction, as losses severely tax weakened defense systems. Theorists and researchers have cited numerous factors that "instigate" neurotic reaction in old age. A partial list of these factors includes: loss of significant objects (Levin, 1965), premorbid personality, decreasing capacity to adapt, concurrent with increasing ego inflexibility (Gitelson, 1948), lack of social support (Holahan and Holahan, 1987), and increasing incidence of narcissistic injuries including changes in appearance, sexual ability, and physical health (Busse, Dovenmuehle, and Brown, 1970). The impact of such circumstances and changes seems undeniable.

SELF-IMAGE IN LATER LIFE

One of the most significant changes that occurs during the later years is the final revision of the self-image, which entails each person's attempt to make an assessment concerning the worth of his/her life (Busse and Pfeiffer, 1977). As a further elaboration of this concept, Erikson (1950) has provided us with a comprehensive developmental life stage model that includes the culminating stage of integrity versus despair. Integrity (or ego integrity) refers to the individual's ability to review life with feelings of satisfaction and minimal regrets. The overall tenor is that of a job well done. Conversely, despair is characterized by feelings of hopelessness and resentment over opportunities missed and promises unfulfilled. From an Eriksonian perspective, failure (despair) in the last life stage is a direct result of unresolved conflicts at earlier life stages. Consequently, Erikson has described his model as having an epigenetic basis in that the successful handling of crises at each successive stage provides a foundation for crisis management in later stages. Epigenesis can also be understood in terms of ego development and functioning since ego strengths and resources allow the individual to handle crises, and success leads to greater ego strength and stability in a pyramid type progression (Sherman, 1981).

SOCIAL BREAKDOWN SYNDROME

Zusman (1966) and Kuypers and Bengtson (1973) have delineated a plausible model of psychological breakdown that pulls together the research and theory we have discussed. Social breakdown syndrome seems to be especially applicable to the elderly. It is a process whereby traumatic events in the social environment interact with deficits in a person's self-concept to produce a downward spiral toward psychological breakdown. On the one hand, deficit in self-concept can most usefully be conceptualized in terms of the Eriksonian framework of unresolved life conflicts leading to weakened ego and self-image (Sherman, 1981). On the other hand, losses are the functional equivalent of traumatic events or difficult transitions which set off the breakdown process. Once in motion, breakdown is further facilitated by preconditions such as physiological deterioration, inadequate social support, and financial instability, which render the individual less able to combat the stress of loss.

The argument for antecedent conditions pointing the way toward psychological breakdown seems logically persuasive. However, some writers contend that the losses and changes attendant to aging (physical alterations, object loss, narcissistic injury) are sufficient in and of themselves to account for neurotic disequilibrium (Blau and Berezin, 1982). In either case, the questions of what types of problems may arise and how they should be treated need to be answered. While an exhaustive listing of late age psychological problems is beyond the scope of this chapter, a review of some of the more prevalent ones will alert the reader to treatment concerns that flow from the peculiar mechanisms underlying neurotic dysfunction in the elderly.

DEPRESSION AND PSYCHONEUROTIC REACTION

The shortcomings of old age, whether physical, social, or psychological, seemingly act to inflate the prevalence of conditions of mild situational depression in aged samples (LaRue, Dessonville, and Jarvik, 1985). Depression, however, is but one facet of a broader category of mental disorder. Psychoneurosis is a wide-ranging malady whose chief characteristic is excessive anxiety of either a conscious or unconscious nature. Although no serious distortion of reality is evident in psychoneurotics, quality of life is nonetheless compromised. Manifestations of psychoneurosis include: mood problems (depression, self-blaming, anxiety), cognitive manifestations (obsessions, negative thoughts, hypochondriacal thoughts, suicidal ideation), and behavior problems such as compulsions

(Busse, Dovenmuehle, and Brown, 1970). The possible influence of medication in producing the above symptoms should always be evaluated in elderly clients (Zarit, Eiler, and Hassinger, 1985).

Finally, the clinician should also be cognizant of the fact that depression is a causative factor in the greater incidence of suicide by the elderly (Zung, 1980; Zeamore and Eames, 1979). Available statistics indicate that the elderly are at greater risk to commit suicide than any other age group (Osgood, 1984). Among the aged, stress is exacerbated by social isolation, loss of role and status (especially for males), and other factors (Townsend, 1968; Osgood, 1984). Miller (1979) states that, for the elderly person, ''self-inflicted death is very much a function of the ability to cope with stress'' (p. 25).

TREATMENT OF PSYCHONEUROSIS

In terms of treatment, it is incumbent upon the therapist to understand how the determinants of psychoneurotic symptomatology in the elderly may differ from other age groups. For example, Busse (1970) has examined the differences in causation of depression for young and elderly adults. He suggests that while introjection of hostile feelings toward others into self is the common basis for situational depression in young adults, such depression in the elderly is more often caused by loss of self-esteem stemming from the individual's inability to meet environmental demands or provide self-security. Failure to meet the demands of environmental press may be caused by decreased efficiency of bodily functions, loss of social roles, financial insecurity, or other factors.

In a similar fashion, Busse has highlighted differences in hypochondriacal reaction (preoccupation with bodily concerns) between young and old adults. Hypochondriacal syndrome in the young is most often brought about by a shift of anxiety over some psychic conflict to a less threatening bodily function. Conversely, in older persons, high bodily concern may be caused by withdrawal from outside interests and/or by a real increase in bodily aches and pains. The recognition of differential causation of hypochondriasis has obvious ramifications for course of treatment undertaken with clients who exhibit this problem. For example, Weinberg (1979) points out that hypochondriacal overconcern in older patients can often be mitigated by frank reeducation regarding the range of activities permissible in the context of diminished physical abilities.

ANXIETY AND ITS TREATMENT

Anxiety is the most distinctive feature of psychoneurosis. Among the elderly, the provocation to be anxious seems to be greater as it is based on the partly accurate assessment that the energy and resources necessary to deal with everyday problems are dwindling. Such assessments may give rise to generalized distorted cognitions (e.g., ''I'm too old to handle this'') in the face of problems (Sherman, 1984).

Anxiety of the type described above is, at least, partly attributable to role loss experienced by the aged. It has been known for some time that role loss is associated with greater introversion and less orientation to the outside world (Neugarten, 1969). Furthermore, Neugarten has also pointed out that role loss makes the aged more passive and less able to perceive themselves as having the stamina necessary to take advantage of opportunities and to overcome obstacles. The usual result of increasing anxiety is decreasing satisfaction with life. At this point, participation in a therapeutic program may become either desirable or necessary. If so, what therapy would be most beneficial?

BEHAVIORAL AND COGNITIVE THERAPIES

In recent years, behavioral and cognitive therapies have been increasingly utilized to ameliorate the psychological stresses and problems faced by different subgroups of the elderly population. This has been brought about by the growing consensus that *intrapsychic therapies* (e.g., psychoanalysis) may be inappropriate for the treatment of older clients. It seems logical that it is counterproductive to reawaken repressed material in elderly patients because there is usually not enough time left to do the reparative work necessary as a result of emotional upheaval caused by disarming the individual (Sherman, 1981). This has created the impetus to seek out other alternatives better suited to the contingencies of later life.

Behavioral therapy seems especially appropriate for use in institutional settings where a more desirable environment may be one combining activities and life-styles that foster independence and decision making (Franks, 1973). In this context, several studies (Hussian and Lawrence, 1978; Hanly, 1981) have shown that rearrangement of operant reward contingencies can help move nursing home clients to become more active and socially responsive. *Cognitive therapies,* on the other hand, seem ideal for use with older people in the community. Ellis and Grieger (1977), in particular, stress the dysfunctional effects of perfectionistic thoughts on self-esteem. The elderly may engage in self-blaming thoughts as the result of reminiscence on past failures. Butler (1975) notes that the elderly almost universally review their lives through active engagement in reminiscence. As such, cognitive therapy (e.g., Rational-Emotive therapy) could be used to restructure damaging self-blaming thoughts which have a negative impact on self-concept. *Rational-Emotive therapy* champions recognition of self-worth on the basis of essential humanity rather than performance (Sherman, 1981) and provides a therapeutic backdrop that is in tune with the realities of old age.

FAMILY THERAPY

Family therapy offers yet another possibility for psychotherapeutic treatment of the elderly. While individual therapy focuses on the intrapsychic and/or interpersonal problems of the aging person, family therapy focuses on the network of relationships in which the person is involved. A family theoretical orientation regards the family as an emotional unit and the symptom in the patient as a product of the total family problem (Carter and McGoldrick, 1980). One of the great contributions of family therapy is its notion of intergenerational connectedness issues and transmission of "family myths." To this end, before intervening with a family, a family therapist obtains information on family membership and significant events in a family over three generations (Guerin, 1976).

In recent years, family therapy has begun to gain greater acceptance by both public agencies and the general public. In terms of family with elderly, it is now not uncommon to find therapy groups that address family-oriented issues such as adult children who care for elderly parents or child rearing in the three-generational family. The real power of the intergenerational approach is that it focuses on problems created by stressors which accumulate over the life span of the family itself.

LEISURE COUNSELING

One therapeutic intervention that may be particularly effective in combating late age anxiety is leisure counseling. Numerous studies have demonstrated that role rejuvenation through participation in leisure pursuits both increases the degree of life satisfaction (Iso-Ahola, 1980) and reduces the impact of life crises, especially after age sixty (DeCarlo, 1974). Counselors should therefore be prepared to explore leisure time activities with their elderly clients. Leisure activities offer the aged a sense of purpose in doing and planning activities for the future. Such future orientation is a critical dimension used by Neugarten and others to measure the extent of life satisfaction.

GOALS FOR THE FUTURE

It has been our objective to define work parameters for the counseling psychologist who deals with the aged. Since there is historical precedence for a disciplinary interest in normative life crises, the posture we have articulated is in the mainstream of what has always been the major thrust of counseling psychology. As with any nascent endeavor, however, our future progress not only depends on our past understandings, but also on our abilities to evolve newer understandings and to build upon emergent trends in service delivery relative to older adult populations. This is especially true since a reversal in the tendency for the elderly to underutilize mental health services in the future may ultimately occur because of increased college attendance today and a resultant psychological sophistication which may translate into a greater willingness to seek assistance without fear of stigmatization. In conclusion, therefore, we suggest the following for consideration. First, at least one study has demonstrated that primary care physicians are often called upon to address the psychological as well as the physical problems of their elderly patients (Goldstrom et al., 1987). This documents, we feel, the lack of resources and mobility among the aged. Consequently, a multidisciplinary consolidation of services in one locus would seem an appropriate professional response to a multiproblem population.

In conjunction with our multiservice orientation, we feel that "visiting the counselor" can become a more routine health maintenance behavior. In this context, prevention and coping become primary operating principles that underlie the delivery of psychological services. The psychologist becomes an educational consultant who facilitates the client's negotiation of normative life crises and provides a bulwark against serious psychological breakdown.

The incidence of the use of cognitive and behavioral therapies with the elderly seems to be on the upswing. Cognitive therapy, in particular, is beneficial in combating the negative thought patterns inherent in the reminiscences of the elderly. As we have previously discussed, the prevalence of anxiety seems to increase with age. It is the authors' view that at least part of this anxiety is a consequence of role loss. This being the case, leisure counseling affords the opportunity of role rejuvenation with its attendant increase in purpose, control, and overall life satisfaction.

CONCLUSION

We have attempted to make the reader aware of the current status of counseling psychology with regard to the elderly. At this point in time, many questions remain unanswered as the field of gerontological counseling psychology is still in its relative infancy. It is the authors' view, however, that the expected and inevitable multiplication in the numbers of elderly will help create a greater professional impetus to resolve these issues. Thus, our understanding of the psychological aspects of aging will undoubtedly expand by virtue of necessity as we enter a twenty-first century populated by a substantially older citizenry.

REFERENCES

Blau, D., and Berezin, M. A. (1982). Neuroses and character disorders. *Journal of Geriatric Psychiatry,* 15, 55–97.

Blazer, D. G. (1982). *Depression in Late Life.* St. Louis: C. V. Mosby.

Blum, J. (1977). Clinical gerontology: A proposed curriculum. In W. D. Gentry (Ed.), *Geropsychology: A Model of Training and Clinical Service,* pp. 127–34. Cambridge, Mass.: Ballinger.

Busse, E. (1970). Psychoneurotic reactions and defense mechanisms in the aged. In E.

Palmore (Ed.), *Normal Aging: Reports from the Duke Longitudinal Study 1955–1969*, pp. 84–90. Durham, N.C.: Duke University Press.

Busse, E., and Pfeiffer, E. (Eds.) (1977). *Behavior and Adaptation in Late Life*. 2d ed. Boston: Little, Brown and Co.

Busse, E., Dovenmuehle, R., and Brown, R. (1970). Psychoneurotic reactions of the aged. In E. Palmore (Ed.), *Normal Aging: Reports from the Duke Longitudinal Study 1955–1969*, pp. 75–83. Durham, N.C.: Duke University Press.

Butler, R. (1975). *Why Survive: Being Old in America*. New York: Harper and Row.

Carter, E., and McGoldrick, M. (1980). *The Family Life Cycle*. New York: Gardner Press.

Cleveland, W. P., and Gianturco, D. T. (1976). Remarriage possibilities after widowhood: A retrospective method. *Journal of Gerontology*, 31, 99–103.

DeCarlo, T. J. (1974). Recreation participation patterns and successful aging. *Journal of Gerontology*, 29, 416–22.

Deutscher, I. (1964). The quality of post-parental life. *Journal of Marriage and Family*, 26, 52–60.

Ellis, A., and Grieger, R. (1977). *Handbook of Rational-Emotive Therapy*. New York: Springer Publishing Co.

Erikson, E. (1950). *Childhood and Society*. New York: Norton.

Fleming, A. S., Buchanan, J. G., Santos, J. F., and Rickards, L. D. (1984). *Mental Health Services for the Elderly: Report on a Survey of Mental Health Centers*. The Action Committee to Implement the Mental Health Recommendations of the 1981 White House Conference on Aging. Washington, D.C.: U.S. Government Printing Office.

Franks, C. (Ed.) (1973). *Annual Review of Behavior Therapy: Theory and Practice*. New York: Brunner/Mazel.

Freud, S. (1924). On psychotherapy. *Collected Papers*. Vol. 1. London: Hogarth Press.

Gitelson, M. (1948). The emotional problems of elderly people. *Geriatrics*, 3, 135–50.

Goldstrom, I. D., Burns, B. J., Kessley, L. G., Feuerberg, M. A., Larson, D. B., Miller, N. E., and Cromer, W. J. (1987). Mental health services use by elderly adults in a primary care setting. *Journal of Gerontology*, 42, 147–53.

Guerin, P. (1976). *Family Therapy: Theory and Practice*. New York: Gardner Press.

Gurland, B. J., and Cross, P. S. (1982). Epidemiology of psychopathology in old age. In L. F. Jarvik and G. W. Small (Eds.), *Psychiatric Clinics of North America*, pp. 11–26. Philadelphia: Saunders.

Hanly, I. (1981). The use of signposts and active training to modify word disorientation in elderly patients. *Journal of Behavior Therapy and Experimental Psychiatry*, 12 (3), 241–47.

Hendricks, J., and Hendricks, C. D. (1986). *Aging in Mass Society: Myths and Realities*. Boston: Little, Brown and Co.

Heyman, D. (1970). Does a wife retire? *Gerontologist*, 10, 54–56.

Holahan, C., and Holahan, C. (1987). Self-efficacy, social support, and depression in aging: A longitudinal analysis. *Journal of Gerontology*, 42, 65–68.

Howells, J. G. (1975). Family psychopathology. In J. G. Howells (Ed.), *Modern Perspectives in the Psychiatry of Old Age*. New York: Brunner/Mazel.

Hussian, R., and Lawrence, P. (1978). The reduction of test, state and trait anxiety by test-specific and generalized stress innoculation training. *Cognitive Therapy and Research*, 2 (1), 25–37.

Iso-Ahola, S. (1980). *The Social Psychology of Leisure and Recreation*. Dubuque, Iowa: Wm. C. Brown Company.

Jung, C. G. (1933). *Modern Man in Search of a Soul*. New York: Harcourt.

Kuypers, J. A., and Bengtson, V. L. (1973). Internal locus of control, ego functioning and personality characteristics in old age. *Gerontologist*, 27, 168–73.

Larsen, D. (1984). *Teaching Psychological Skills: Model for Giving Psychology Away*. Monterey, Calif.: Brooks Cole.

LaRue, A., Dessonville, C., and Jarvik, L. F. (1985). Aging and mental disorders. In J. E. Birren and K. W. Schaie (Eds.), *Handbook of the Psychology of Aging*. 2d ed., pp. 664–92. New York: Van Nostrand Reinhold.

Levin, S. (1965). Depression in the aged. In M. A. Berezin and S. H. Cath (Eds.), *General Psychiatry: Grief, Loss, and Emotional Disorders in the Aging Process*, pp. 203–25. New York: International University Press.

Maslow, A. H. (1954). *Motivation and Personality*. New York: Harper.

Miller, M. (1979). *Suicide after Sixty: The Final Alternative*. New York: Springer.

Neugarten, B. L. (1969). Continuities and discontinuities of psychological issues into adult life. *Human Development*, 12, 121–30.

Neugarten, B. L. (1970). Dynamics of transition from middle age to old age: Adaptation and the life cycle. *Journal of Geriatric Psychiatry*, 4, 71–87.

Neugarten, B. L., and Weinstein, K. (1968). The changing American grandparent. In B. Neugarten (Ed.), *Middle Age and Aging*. Chicago: University of Chicago Press.

Osgood, N. J. (1984). Suicides. In E. Palmore (Ed.), *Handbook on the Aged in the United States*. Westport, Conn.: Greenwood Press.

Osgood, N. J., and McIntosh, J. (1986). *Suicide and the Elderly: An Annotated Bibliography and Review*. Westport, Conn.: Greenwood Press.

Redick, R. W., Kramer, M., and Taube, C. A. (1973). Epidemiology of mental illness and utilization of psychiatric facilities among older persons. In E. W. Busse and E. Pfeiffer (Eds.), *Mental Illness in Later Life*. Washington, D.C.: American Psychiatric Association.

Rollins, B., and Feldman, H. (1970). Marital satisfaction over the family life cycle. *Journal of Marriage and Family*, 32, 20–28.

Schurman, R. A., Kramer, P. D., and Mitchell, J. B. (1985). The hidden mental health network. *Archives of General Psychiatry*, 42, 89–94.

Shanas, E., and Maddox, G. L. (1985). Health, health resources and the utilization of counseling. In E. Shanas and G. L. Maddox (Eds.), *Handbook of Aging and the Social Sciences*. 2d ed., pp. 696–726. New York: Van Nostrand Reinhold.

Sherman, E. (1981). *Counseling the Aging*. New York: The Free Press.

Sherman, E. (1984). *Working with Older Persons—Cognitive and Phenomenological Methods*. Boston: Kluwer-Nijhoff.

Stenmark, D. E., and Dunn, V. K. (1982). Issues related to the training of geropsychologists. In J. F. Santos and G. R. VandenBos (Eds.), *Psychology and the Older Adult*, pp. 83–96. Washington, D.C.: American Psychological Association.

Storandt, M. (1983). Psychology's response to the graying of America. *American Psychologist*, 38 (3), 323–26.

Townsend, P. (1968). Isolation, desolation and loneliness. In E. Shanas, P. Townsend,

H. Wedderburn, P. Milhof, and G. Stehouwer (Eds.), *Old People in Three In-dustrial Societies*. New York: Atherton Press.

U.S. Department of Health, Education and Welfare, Federal Council on Aging. (1979). *Mental Health and the Elderly: Recommendations for Action*. Washington, D.C.: DHEW Publication No. 80–209607.

Weinberg, J. (1979). Psychopathology. In J. Hendricks and C. Hendricks (Eds.), *Dimensions in Aging*, pp. 160–71. Cambridge, Mass.: Winthrop Publishers.

Weissman, M. M., Myers, J. K., Tischler, G. L., Holzer, C. E., III, Leaf, P. J., Or-uashel, H., and Brody, J. A. (1985). Psychiatric disorders (DSM III) and cognitive impairment among the elderly in a U.S. urban community. *Acta Psychiatrica Scandinavica*, 71, 366–79.

Williams, R., Jr. (1970). *American Society*. New York: Alfred A. Knopf.

Zarit, S. H., Eiler, J., and Hassinger, M. (1985). Clinical assessment. In J. Birren and K. W. Schaie (Eds.), *Handbook of the Psychology of Aging*. 2d ed., pp. 725–54. New York: Van Nostrand Reinhold.

Zeamore, R., and Eames, N. (1979). Psychic and somatic symptoms of depression among young adults, institutionalized aged, and noninstitutionalized aged. *Journal of Gerontology*, 34, 716–22.

Zung, W. (1980). Affective disorders. In E. Busse and D. Blazer (Eds.), *Handbook of Geriatric Psychology*. New York: Van Nostrand Reinhold.

Zusman, J. (1966). Some explanations of the changing appearance of psychotic patients: Antecedents of the social breakdown syndrome concept. *The Milbank Memorial Fund Quarterly*, 64, 363–94.

8. SOCIAL WORK AND AGING

Louis Lowy

> The role of theory is crucial because it guides the interpretation and explanation of experience, information and observation and it assists in anticipating the future.
>
> David McMaldonado, Jr., 1986, p. 103

CURRENT TRENDS IN THEORY, RESEARCH, AND PRACTICE OF SOCIAL WORK WITH THE AGING

Despite the fact that in the last thirty years a great deal has become known about aging as a bio-psycho-social-cultural phase in the human life span, relatively little has been offered in the way of explaining and understanding the processes of aging. To be sure, there exist a sizable number of theories: biological, psychological, economic, sociological, anthropological, etc., that fill the increasing shelves of gerontologic literature. Many of these theories are addressed in other chapters of this volume. As aging affects the whole person in his/her situation and environment, social work as a discipline and as a field of practice is closely linked with gerontology. The following framework delineates social work as a profession and as a field of practice within a societal matrix. This framework consists of five components: values, purposes, sanctions, knowledge, and intervention.

Two major sets of *values* have formed the normative foundation of the profession: (1) the worth, dignity, and uniqueness of the individual person, of families, of groups and constituents in a community. These values are helpful guidelines in resisting negative stereotypes, promoting independence and assertiveness among the aging, and advocating for the basic rights of the elderly (Lowy, 1985). (2) the responsibility of society to create equitable social and economic justice and with social security as a foundation to ensure a decent standard of living for all people at any phase in their lives.

The interactions of these two major value-sets are the bedrock upon which the *purposes* of social work are built. They span a continuum from treatment to development; they are curative and ameliorative as well as preventive and pro-motional/enhancing. Older persons, singly, in families or groups, at home or in institutions, face intra- and interpersonal tensions and stress, as do also younger people; however, among the elderly these tensions are frequently aggravated by deteriorating health conditions and increasing losses against diminishing gains. Older people face status and role conflicts, age-connected isolation, many times economic hardships, and, not infrequently, generational conflicts. Hence the *purposes* of social work include: (1) to help older people enlarge their competence and increase their problem-solving and coping abilities; (2) to help the elderly obtain necessary resources; (3) to make organizations responsive to older people; (4) to facilitate interaction between individuals and others in their environment; (5) to influence interactions between organizations and institutions; and (6) to influence social and environmental social policy (Monk, 1981).

Social work is *sanctioned* by society as a field of practice and as a profession. Settings and auspices in which social workers carry out their activities in a community, city, or county, on the state or on federal levels vary considerably, depending on the objectives and orientations of programs and services offered (Bartlett, 1970).

There are formal and informal programs and services. "Public policy in the last fifty years has responded unevenly to the demographic imperatives of an aging society," says Elaine Brody (1986). The two major *public* policy mech-anisms under federal governmental auspices are (1) the Older Americans Act, initially passed in 1965 and amended several times and reauthorized, and (2) the Social Security Act, whose origin dates back to 1935 with many amendments, changes, and adaptations since that time. It is the major foundation block of our public social policy; it is our society's major response to the economic needs of our aging population (Schottland, 1970). Within this space one cannot do justice to the complexities of this piece of national legislation that presently affects over 36 million Americans. It suffices to point out that the social insurance part of the Social Security Act (Title II) is essentially income-related and provides a minimum floor of cash payments to employees, workers, and the self-employed beginning at age sixty-two. It also includes disability insurance and benefits for survivors and dependents of insured workers. In 1965 Medicare (Title XVIII), an age-categorical health insurance program, providing hospital coverage under Part A and Supplemental Medical Insurance under Part B for ambulatory care, was added for retirees. For the indigent patient Medicaid (Title XIX) was enacted. Social insurance and Medicare are primarily financed through compulsory con-tributions from employers, employees, and the self-employed. Medicaid is ex-clusively supported through tax funds. Because of the tremendous increase in financial outlays with a burgeoning aging population, the Social Security program financing and benefit mechanisms were restructured in 1983.

In 1988 the largest single expansion of Medicare's twenty-three years was legislated, the Catastrophic Health Care Bills, to provide coverage for catastrophic illness, notably extended nursing home stays. It will be phased in beginning January 1, 1989, through January 1, 1991. However, for the first time in Medicare's history the enrollees, the elderly themselves, will be expected to pay for the entire benefits program. Despite these adaptations the Social Security Act is by no means an adequate instrument to meet the financial and fiscal health needs of our aging population. The comparatively small number of private pension plans of corporations, industry, trade unions, and other organizations are equally insufficient to supplement the economic shortfall adequately.

The elderly are in particular need of long-term medical and mental health care; that is where our public programs have particularly fallen short. We are still "cure" rather than "care" oriented. In contrast to acute illnesses, chronic ailments require many more supportive health and social services in addition to medical and medically related treatment (Huttman, 1985).

In addition, mental and emotional illnesses are highly correlated with physical disease (Goldfarb, 1965; Birren and Sloane, 1980). Indeed, the mental health picture of the elderly population is rather dismal, and the increase of Alzheimer's disease (or at least the awareness of its encroachment upon older persons) has created concern and despair among many families (*Journal of Gerontological Social Work*, 1985–1986).

The Older Americans Act of 1965, amended again in 1986, establishes program objectives and federal/state funding to plan, administer, and provide selected social services to meet social needs of citizens sixty years of age and older. It consists of seven titles, of which Title III is probably the most significant, as it is the principal source of funding via state and county governments to plan and provide social services. The overall federal agency dealing administratively with the Act is the Administration on Aging in the U.S. Department of Health and Human Services. In every state there are a number of area agencies on aging, i.e., regional centers, which under a designated state agency receive funding to carry out its approved state plan, administer and develop social service programs, such as information-referral services, home care programs, respite services, volunteer services, educational programs, chore and homemaker services, etc. Depending on locality and organization, the "triple-A" agencies (presently there are over 500 in the country) vary in size, effectiveness, efficiency, operational capability, and types of service delivery. There are no uniform national standards. On top, the fiscal underpinning of the Act is kept rather low and precarious and therefore many communities suffer from a serious lack of services as well as a lack of coordination of those services that do exist (Huttman, 1985; Monk, 1985).

In addition to these formal policy mechanisms there is an *informal* system of programs and services that has preceeded the public, formal sector since the 1920s. And today, the informal system is still the main source of social assistance, providing at least 80 percent of the health/social services received by the elderly (U.S. General Accounting Office, 1987). Together, the public and private sectors constitute what has come to be known as the "aging network," particularly since the 1971 White House Conference on Aging (1971), the second of its kind in the United States (Estes, 1979).

The third source of programs and services stems from the organized elderly population itself, such as the American Association of Retired Persons (AARP) with a membership of close to 3 million elderly, the Gray Panthers, linking old and young as an activist organization, the National Caucus and Center of the Black Aged, the National Council of Senior Citizens, Center for Understanding Aging, Generations United Together for Tomorrow, and many, many more. Huttman provides a useful typology of "Service Provisions" according to "Needs and Programs," such as economic needs, food and nutrition, shelter/ housing, transportation and mobility needs, health-related needs, and social contact/leisure needs. Further classifications of her matrix are provided along the following dimensions: income and health status of users; locale of service; type of service and type of sponsors. These classifications may have emerged as a result of policy decisions as the best way to provide a service, or they may have simply been historical accidents (Huttman, 1985). It is important, however, to keep in mind that despite the reference to an "aging network," it is more a patchwork of programs and services that do not meet the criteria of universality, continuous availability, and coordinated, comprehensive accessibility.

Through its major professional organization, the National Association of Social Workers (NASW), the profession of social work has set up a number of councils, commissions, task forces, and committees to focus on the special needs of the aging, on their relationship to the middle and younger generations, to social work practice with individuals, family members, peer groups, short- and long-term care facilities, hospices, home caring efforts by adult children, mental health counseling and therapy, case management, and caring for the homeless and impoverished single elderly.

In 1983, the Council on Social Work Education (CSWE) developed a project to expand and strengthen the capabilities of schools of social work to prepare practitioners and to train students on the master's and baccalaureate levels to work more effectively and cogently with an increasingly larger elderly population. Several curricular models have been designed and an appreciable number are being applied in the 93 graduate and over 250 undergraduate schools or departments. Increasing emphasis is placed on collaborative efforts with other disciplines and fields (public health, human services, nursing, allied health, education, etc.) to help students acquire value orientations that counteract "ageism" in any form, and to learn to perform organizational and planning management tasks in the public and private sectors of social gerontology (Lowy, 1985).

The *knowledge base* of social work with the aging is manifold and eclectic.

It draws heavily on information, theoretical propositions, and hypotheses that have been developed in the social sciences, in the fields of geriatrics and gerontology, notably: biophysiological data and knowledge related to the skeletal and muscular systems, to the circulatory, endocrine, respiratory, and nervous systems, as well as to the digestive and reproductive systems and to the functioning of the five senses. But social work, given its goals and functions, is more familiar and conversant with cognitive, affective, behavioral, and learning patterns and various personality theories that the field of social gerontology utilizes in its search for its theoretical underpinnings. Disengagement and activity theories, subculture and life satisfaction theories, continuity and exchange theories, social breakdown, stratification and developmental theories have found their way into gerontological social work. Psychodynamic (Freudian, Jungian, e.g.) stances have by no means been neglected, although Eriksonian and ego-theoretical frameworks have found readier adherents in social work practice with the aging (Monk, 1985; Lowy, 1985; Meyer, 1986; Atchley, 1977; Brody, 1986).

Increasingly, attention has been given to phase theories with their emphasis upon developmental tasks in the later years which themselves undergo varying stages of development, from the onset of aging phenomena to managing the stages of dying (e.g., Lowenthal, Chiroboza, and Thurnber, 1975). McClusky's theory of "Margins of Power" (1971), which postulates that older people frequently face a disruption in their sense of autonomy because of an increase in their load (e.g., increased expenses, new caregiving responsibilities, illness, role losses, demands on energy, loss of income and status, etc.), has found many adherents who argue for increasing power to the aged by reducing their loads (e.g., through services and educational or other type activities via community programs).

Recently social workers have been more in search of micromodels rather than micro- or macrotheories. Building on Germain/Gitterman's "Life Model," Lowy (1985) proposes the "Life Model for the Aging." He points out that aging is a form of life-transitional processes. When getting older (say sixty-five to seventy or eighty to eighty-five and beyond) specific crises and exigencies occur in people's lives that require personal adaptations and coping with such events. Environmental situational conditions both physical and social, natural crises and disasters, dealing with bureaucratic structures and organizations (e.g., Social Security offices), or negotiating the ins and outs of the "aging network" (e.g., obtaining entitlements) posit tasks that older people, singly or in groups, need to be able to handle in order to "make it." Complex patterns of interpersonal relationships and communications in family and peer relationships, disturbances in communications with kin, friends, officials, functionaries, physicians, mental health counselors, social workers, educators, etc., permeate the day-to-day functioning of people. As they grow older and their strengths and personal resources diminish (even if they belong to the group of the healthy aged), persons in their later years are increasingly faced with these demands and have a tougher time coping with the imbalance in the relationship between person and society.

Eyde and Rich, in their "Family Management Model," base their approach on the "family-as-a-unit" concept and look at the older person from the Gestalt perspective (Eyde and Rich, 1983). They suggest that relationships are influenced by the structural and communication patterns of the family group. By encouraging analytic understanding of behavioral interactive patterns this model attempts to alleviate dysfunctional family patterns and promotes functional behaviors by educating members and altering structural arrangements of the family.

Silverstone and Burack-Weiss (1983) describe the "Auxiliary Function Model" which also looks at the family as a basic unit of social functioning rather than the individual, but assigns to social work the task of supplementing the roles that family members or significant others cannot perform.

Greene (1986a, 1986b) presents the "Functional Age Model" of intergenerational theory that is to provide social work with a systemic family approach. It is concerned with both the elderly person's functioning and the family system in which it takes place. Based on the psychosocial model of social casework it adds two aspects: the importance of sufficiently addressing the biological aspects of the aging process and the need to encourage family participation in treatment. As Greene points out, "It should be acknowledged, however, that the goal of closing the gap between social work theory and social work practice is difficult to achieve. It involves the integration of the most current knowledge of human behavior and the adaptation of existing methods and techniques" (Greene, 1986a, p. 2).

Despite these shortcomings in theory and model building, the efforts of the social sciences and the applied fields, such as social work, to engage in empirical research (quantative and qualitative) are rushing along with unabated speed. The growth in the literature within the last ten years is astounding and, what is more, gerontological social work not only makes use of theories and research in the social sciences, but is busily engaged in designing its own theoretical constructs and research undertakings toward achieving a better understanding of the aging process in order to be more effective in its intervention repertoire. (A cursory review of the articles in *The Gerontologist* or in the *Journal of Gerontological Social Work* provides ample documentation.)

The fifth component of social work practice is the *intervention process,* the action of the practitioner that is directed to some part of social systems (individual, family, group, community, agency, organization) or social processes (interpersonal relationships) and educational activities with the intention of inducing a change in them (Lowy, 1974; Siporin, 1975).

Historically, intervention has involved social work methods of casework (working with individuals and their social network), group work (working with groups of people and their affiliates), and community organization (working with community groups, members of neighborhoods, social action to effect changes of the immediate environment to improve social conditions). It is through the goal-directed, systematic activities of the social worker, who selects what is relevant to deal with a particular situation, that appropriate knowledge and values become integrated and change is sought and not infrequently achieved (Compton and Galaway, 1975).

Presently these "classical methods" have been superseded by utilizing new interventive repertoires—often based on "social systems"' theories—that can be adapted to meet specific needs and resolve particular problems or, if possible, prevent these problems from occurring in the first place (Pincus and Monahan, 1972; Compton and Galaway, 1975; Shulman, 1986).

Social workers, after making as full an assessment (diagnosis) of the condition or situation as possible (primarily along psycho-social-cultural lines without neglecting biological and physical functioning), formulate specific goals for what to do about these conditions or situations. Most significant in this effort is the nature and type of mutual professional relationship between worker and client through which assessment and goal formulation are accomplished. Based upon mutually agreed upon goals in working with individuals or group members, worker and client embark upon social treatment when social functioning is impaired (e.g., when an older person or a group of older people, including families, experience problems of psychological dysfunctioning, when they feel isolated or under stress). Social workers provide care management at home or in an institution when and where aged persons can't cope with their daily tasks, linking persons, family members, peers, and agencies whenever needed. They offer recreational and educational services to enhance self-realization and encourage social participation and action (Steinberg and Carter, 1983). Social workers also engage in advocacy with and on behalf of their constituents to achieve social changes in a neighborhood or community.

The emergence of the "life model" has significantly contributed to these reconceptualizations of the interventive stance, as it promulgates a holistic social systems view. Particularly, the comprehensiveness and systemic nature of the aging process make social work a key form of professional practice. Social work, in its value orientations, its holistic approach, and its linkage functions, is ideally suited to provide services to the elderly. When action is required to make changes in the social milieu (e.g., in income—Social Security, in health care—Medicare, in housing arrangements, in bringing young and old together, etc.) social work's skills in social action and advocacy are as essential as its skills of intra- and interpersonal counseling.

In the intervention process there are four major steps: selecting specific targets (clients), focusing on goals, engaging in interventive activities of the social work jointly with the client through appropriate methods and techniques, and utilizing the intervener in his/her roles as enabler (facilitator), broker, advocate, expert, therapist, and teacher. The steps of intervention are schematically highlighted in Figure 8.1.

WHAT ARE THE PRESENT FRONTIERS OF RESEARCH IN SOCIAL WORK WITH THE AGING?

The following selective listing of topics provides some answers to this question:

1. Demographic patterns and their impact upon the United States and world society, particularly with regard to changing family structures, physical, mental, and emotional health services, housing arrangements, and economic conditions

Figure 8.1
Representation of "Life-Model" and Intervention Processes of Social Work

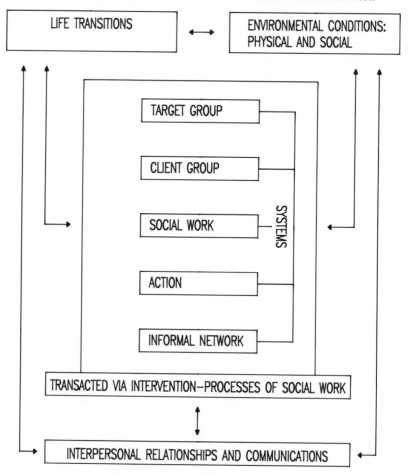

Source: Louis Lowy, *Social Work with the Aging*, 2d edition. New York: Longman, Inc., 1985.
              Reprinted by permission.

2. Parental relationships and their influence upon filial maturity

3. Intergenerational relationships and their impact on caregiving

4. Care (case) management and its effect upon caregivers and carereceivers

5. Housing arrangements for the acute and chronically ill elderly, as well as for the well elderly

6. Economic conditions and their relationship to the daily living of people in their later years

7. Independence, dependence, and interdependence of older persons

8. Widow- and widowerhood; impact upon their lives and those in their environment

9. Minority group characteristics of the aged and their status in American society

10. The relationships of the aging "enterprise" to the aging "network"

11. Intergenerational equity and the political power of the aged

12. Education by, for, with the elderly

13. Coping with dying, bereavement, and grief

14. The future of Social Security and pension plans

15. Planning for an aging society in the political, economic, and social sectors of our society

16. Age or need? The direction of public policies toward older people

17. Grandparenthood as part of the life cycle

18. Alzheimer's disease and related chronic disorders and their impact upon family and friends

19. Elder abuse and its effects upon abuser and victim

While appreciable research undertakings in social work with the aging are under way all over the country, most of them are conducted under the auspices of academic institutions, by national organizations, and federal/state and local governments. Smaller agencies (public or private) are not infrequently part of such enterprises, but they do not constitute the majority of the sponsors. Samples generally are quite small and frequently are a "captive population," since subjects are sought and found in institutional settings. Despite the fact that results of studies are presented at many local, regional, and national conferences and that there are an increasing number of gerontological journals reporting social work research, and that these types of activities proliferate at an exponential rate, there is very little effort under way to coordinate the results of such investigations, to pick up "unfinished business," or to design major longitudinal studies of specifically selected topics or themes. To be sure, in recent years more data on fewer topics have been accumulated and more replications of studies done earlier have yielded more reliable results that offer glimpses of social work's involvement with the elderly and also document a certain degree of effectiveness to meet some of their needs and deal with some of their problems. However, the well elderly, those who show strengths, zest, and continuing engagement in the lives of their immediate surrounding world, are among the least-researched group of older people; as a result we know little about them, except that economic well-being and good physical and mental health (often correlated) present a solid foundation for a "good old age" (Comfort, 1976). We are still quite uninformed why certain types of older people cope more successfully with their losses than others, why they can deal better with retirement from work, why they accept aging as a "normal stage of life," rather than an inevitable decline, enjoy grandparenthood more and feel included in their communities rather than excluded in society. We begin to have some understanding why caregiving by and for the elderly has varied meanings to them and their families, why cultural and spiritual aspects assume different significance for some groups of elderly, why urban, suburban, and rural elderly hold different expectations, and why many people who have been discriminated against throughout their lives—whether because of gender, color, ethnicity, or class—find old age to be a period of despair rather than integrity.

The debate about quantitative and qualitative research is as lively in social work as it is in the social sciences, though it is recognized that knowledge-building and its verification requires both types of research. Analysis of intra-personal interviews, observations of behavior in long-term care institutions by staff and residents, examination of receptivity of the elderly to services by community agencies, or by kin and friends, studies of attitudes of the young, the middle-aged, and the old regarding the process of aging, as well as the aged themselves, are rich sources for quantitative and ethnomethodological data collections that can shed a good deal of light on the way in which social workers can contribute to improving the life-style and living conditions of people in their later years.

HISTORICAL ROOTS

The first bibliographic references in social work with the aging appear in 1926 in a paper entitled, "Provision for care of the aged" by the Russell Sage Foundation (see Lowy, 1985, *Social Work with the Aging,* Chapter 2: "Historical Notes on Social Work with the Aging").

Despite the emergence in this century of a sizable aging population with concomitant social, medical, and economic problems, there was no significant professional or public interest in this demographic phenomenon until the early 1930s among the general population, among social scientists, and social workers (*Social Work Yearbook,* 1949). In 1930 the Deutsch Foundation sponsored a conference on care of the aged (Rubinow, 1930), and in 1937 the New York Committee on Mental Hygiene of the Family Welfare Association of America provided a series of weekly lectures for professionals working with the aged, which culminated in the publication of *Mental Hygiene in Old Age (Social Work Yearbook,* 1949).

Increased attention to the elderly was fostered by the founding of the Gerontological Society in 1945, which began publication of the *Journal of Gerontology* and *The Gerontologist,* which ever since have remained major periodicals in the field (Gerontological Society of America, 1945).

At the National Conference of Social Workers in 1947 Rose McHugh spoke of "a constructive program for the aged," and Raymond Hillard stressed the causes of dependency and chronic illness in old age rather than the treatment of symptoms (National Conference of Social Workers, 1947 Proceedings).

In the 1949 *Social Work Yearbook* Ruth Hill described a beginning interest in the welfare of older people by voluntary social agencies but also admitted to the lack of a body of experience in casework with the aged. Schools of social work did not offer any special courses, though there were a small number of field placements (internships) in social agencies serving older people.

In 1952, social workers spoke of the reluctance of family service agencies to work with the elderly. However, group work as a method proved useful in bringing older people together in the community and was instrumental in creating senior centers in settlement houses (the first was the Hodson Center in New York City), community centers, YMCAs and YWCAs, neighborhood houses, and in homes for the aged (Kubie and Landau, 1953).

In *The Needs of Older People and Public Welfare Services to Meet Them,* Elizabeth Wickenden (1953) discusses the effects of changing family patterns, industrialization, and the lengthening life span and bemoans the lack of commitment to the care of the aged by social welfare agencies and social workers.

In the mid-fifties Helen Turner and William Posner pioneered casework services to the elderly (*Social Casework,* 1954). Not until 1958 was there a major breakthrough; however, the Council on Social Work Education, the accrediting body of schools of social work, with support from the Ford Foundation, the Public Welfare Association, and the National Institute of Mental Health, sponsored a landmark Seminar on Aging in Aspen, Colorado (1958). It provided model curricula for schools of social work and initiated collaborative efforts by practitioners and educators to develop field instruction opportunities with aging clients, to produce teaching materials, and also made a limited number of scholarships available to master's degree students of social work in order to encourage recruitment to the field.

Leadership by the National Council on Aging in 1960 grew out of a "Committee on Aging" initiated by the National Social Welfare Assembly. The Council, jointly with social work professional organizations, sponsored seminars with published proceedings on *Casework with the Aging, Social Groups with Older People,* and *Community Organizing and Planning for Older Adults.*

The first White House Conference on Aging in 1961 set the tone for increasing federal involvement in serving the elderly, and John F. Kennedy's historic address in 1963, "The Elderly Citizens of Our Nation," can be viewed as a milestone in the initiation of public policy toward older people in this country.

After these turning points, the social work profession started a number of jointly sponsored projects with the National Institute of Mental Health, the National Jewish Welfare Board, the Central Bureau for the Jewish Aged, the Family Service Association, the American Public Welfare Association, and a host of other national organizations, as well as schools of social work, to promote social work practice with the elderly. Senior centers continued to grow (in the 1960s there were over 500 and in the early 1980s over 8,000 were listed by the National Council on Aging). The Heller School at Brandeis University was the first academic institution to develop a specialization in aging, however only on the doctoral level; soon after, it was followed by master's programs at Boston University, New York University, Wayne State, State University of New York, and the University of Michigan, to name a few.

Some of the policy resolutions of the 1971 White House Conference on Aging, buttressed by a growing self-awareness of the aging themselves as a viable political force, found their way into national legislation. The aged had become visible and, as a group of conscientious voters, had to be reckoned with. "Senior Power" became more than a slogan (Hudson, 1981).

During the seventies, curriculum building in schools of social work (and other schools, such as public health, nursing) continued on a more sophisticated level. The gap between theory and practice became more apparent; politicians, economists, sociologists, in addition to physicians, dentists, nurses, the clergy, and social workers as well as leaders in industry, corporations, and labor began to realize the demographic shifts and their implications.

It was not until 1974 that the National Association of Social Workers established a Council on Social Work Services to the Aging, and in 1980 the *Journal of Gerontological Social Work* appeared for the first time on the scene. In 1982 the Council on Social Work Education cosponsored the National Council on Aging's annual meeting and in 1982 the Gerontological Society of America featured a session, "Social Work Practice: Unique Contributions to Programs and Services to the Aged." The organized social work profession, the Council on Social Work Education, schools of social work, and national, regional, and state social welfare organizations have paid greater attention to the aging as a significant part of the population and have geared many of their programs to meeting several of their needs. Aging had come of age! After the politically controversial 1981 White House Conference and despite the new fiscal conservatism in the Reagan administration, a number of programs, notably Social Security, have been maintained, though cuts in substantial social allocations (and consequently in services) have been a serious setback to the poorer, low-income elderly and also to many middle-class elderly.

Indeed, a backlash against the "graying of the federal budget" has occurred and a sector of society maintains there is allegedly an inequity in our social policy favoring the elderly versus the young, an allegation that has been steadily refuted.

Despite efforts in social work to infuse aging content into social work curricula and to increase practice opportunities for learning, and despite recruitment efforts to attract students and faculty, gerontological social work has not become overly popular as a field of choice (Nelson and Schneider, 1984). To be sure, there are over 5 percent of all Master of Social Work students enrolled in "gerontological social work" (Nelson and Schneider, 1984), an appreciable increase since the 1970s, but they still constitute only a minority of all concentrators. It is important to point out that even those who opt for other service concentrations—alcoholism, 2.4 percent; family services, 13.6 percent; health, 15.0 percent; mental health, 24.2 percent—nolens volens are involved with elderly clients and/or their family members. Therefore it is difficult to say how many social workers are really being trained at the M.S.W. level to work with the elderly. Unquestionably, as in other professions, more and more practitioners face people in their later years, and the problem lies in the lack of systematic preparation attitudinally as well as on the knowledge and skill levels to deal and work with the aging population. Self-help groups call on social workers to give them a headstart or to act as consultants to them. Agencies and private practitioners actively seek gerontological consultation. Policymakers, planners, and administrators are faced with new phenomena for which they have not been adequately prepared.

As already pointed out, research activities, while on an ascending curve in social work in general, devote a relatively small proportion of their efforts to gerontological problems. Even rarer are those studies that address such questions: What makes for successful aging? How can the later years be filled with meaningful content? What new time rhythms get established when people retire from work, childrearing, and household management? How can creativity be fostered and nurtured as people get older?

FUTURE FRONTIER AND UNADDRESSED ISSUES

As we leave the eighties and move into the end of the twentieth century with a puzzling look at what is in store in the year 2000, the demographic revolution with its myriad consequences is one of the most significant factors to shape our destiny in the world. Unless madness overtakes man and womankind and we move toward Armaggedon, the demographic implications point to three- and four-generation households, families, or living units, whatever the actual arrangements may be called.

- How will the public and private sectors collaborate to help employees with aging parents meet the often competing demands of families and work?
- How will our society provide housing and economic and social support for a large percentage of the population, many of them alone, frail, and economically dependent?
- How will we restructure our health care and health-care delivery systems so that quality medical and social care will be available to all who need it?
- With the traditional view that the elderly are no longer capable or useful, how will our economic and social institutions accommodate an ever-growing number of elderly who do not want to retire, but are still healthy, active, and productive?
- How can intergenerational equity be maintained and reciprocal transactions between the young, the middle-aged, and the elderly be achieved?
- What educational, recreational opportunities can be created for older people that bring them into contact with other age groups and yet also preserve their own prerogatives and meet their needs based on biopsychological, social, cultural, and spiritual qualities unique at this stage in life?

Let me single out issues in four arenas: the family, social welfare policy, social work practice, and the social work profession.

1. *The Family*. Presently, an estimated 75 percent of the old remain in independent living situations, cared for by spouses of either sex, while 18 percent live with an adult child. There are relatively few older people living in isolation;

80 percent of the elderly see a close relative every week (*The State of Families,* 1984–1985). Because of the increase of older people who are dependent upon health and social care supports, the prospect is of an aging population in which the old will be caring for the very old—with all the emotional and financial strains which that implies. Right now, at least 5 million Americans are caring for a parent on any given day and, for all their dedication to the task, they experience profound stress in the process. What is needed is some orchestration of assistance to the elderly and to the caregivers to alleviate this stress. Just look at those families who have to care for persons suffering from Alzheimer's disease and have joined numerous mutual aid/self-help groups *(Journal of Gerontological Social Work,* 1985–1986).

Family relationships of older persons are maintained through a system of exchange of resources and services. Help is provided across generations by older persons receiving as well as giving help. The majority of elders also help their spouses, children, and grandchildren; they also receive help from their spouses and children, such as assistance with home repairs, housework, babysitting, care in illness, and various kinds of gifts. Many older people function as vital, contributing members of the family. They do not only obtain needed resources from their children, they also reciprocate as much as their means allow. Adult children and grandchildren benefit from their parents' contributions at the same time as the elderly themselves gain from the help they receive from their children. The ability of older persons to give as well as to receive within the family network is an important contribution to the maintenance of the self-esteem of the elderly.

In October 1988 the First National Conference on Intergenerational Issues and Programs was held in Washington, D.C. The executive directors of the Child Welfare League of America and the National Council on the Aging had formed a coalition—"Generations United"—in 1986 to highlight intergenerational issues affecting people of *all* ages in order to unite our public policy efforts in the area of common issues faced by Americans of every generation and promote programs that increase intergenerational cooperation and exchange.

2. *Social Welfare Policy and Social Services.* The social insurance system that has grown up in this country since 1935 was a major new departure—financial as well as philosophical—committing the federal government to care for its vulnerable citizens. In 1986 the total benefits from these programs inched beyond the $200 million mark. The growth in federal transfer payments to the elderly is the primary reason for a decline in the poverty rate among the elderly. Medicare has seen its budget grow from $5.8 billion in 1970 to an estimated $71.8 billion today. Thirty-six million elderly and disabled people now take part in the federally financed health insurance program (Binstock, 1986).

Because of its soaring costs, Medicare, in particular, has become a prime target of the Reagan administration's budget cutters; since 1981 Congress has agreed to cutbacks worth more than $18 billion through a series of changes aimed at hospitals, doctors, and beneficiaries alike. Pressure for further cuts in Medicare spending has been intensified by reports of looming bankruptcy of the program's hospital insurance trust fund. Despite the reforms of 1983, the "date of doom" has been pushed back from the late 1980s to the late 1990s.

The Social Security program is an "intergenerational transfer program," as the younger generation takes care of the older generation through a national administrative mechanism. Will Social Security survive? Though opinions differ as to why, the consensus is overwhelmingly yes. It has public and political support, because, as a social insurance program, it has proved to be a good arrangement for providing a predictable retirement-income benefit linked with work productivity, while at the same time respecting the dignity of the individual beneficiary.

As of the fall of 1988 the following data have been released by the chair of the Subcommittee on Social Security:

• The Social Security Trust Fund is growing at $109,440,000 per day. This comes to $1 billion every ten days!

• The Reserve will reach $100 billion at the end of the year.

• It will reach $1.4 trillion by the year 2000. This is the equivalent of the present value of all private pension plans.

• By 2005, it will reach $4.5 trillion. (Senator Daniel Patrick Moynihan, Private Communication, September 1988.)

We have abolished mandatory retirement, but the key in the future is to adjust our Social Security system to create options to establish "flexible retirement" patterns and equitability for men and women. The Older Americans Act is the only federal piece of legislation exclusively directed to the social care of the elderly; however, it needs to be strengthened, fiscally and programmatically.

The price of family caregiving can be high. That is why *respite care* is essential to alleviate stress to avoid situations that may lead to "elder abuse," a topic much in the news and yet little understood, despite a number of empirical studies. While pathological factors seem to account for a good deal of abusive behavior, it cannot be overlooked that caring for aging family members, particularly those who suffer from incurable and deteriorating diseases such as Alzheimer's, places enormous emotional, social, and economic burdens upon caregivers. Respite care is one arrangement to reduce such burden and stress. Respite care either offers a substitute care provider to allow family members to "get a respite" from caretaking or makes it possible for the older person to spend a few days or weeks away from the family to enjoy a vacation. The former service option of respite care is increasingly being offered in a number of states. Massachusetts has started to implement such a program through its decentralized system of twenty-seven Homecare Corporations (Massachusetts Executive Office of Elder Affairs, 1984 Annual Report).

Of particular significance has been and continues to be the development of *hospices* as service for persons who have been diagnosed as terminally ill. It focuses on the personal well-being of the dying individual, aiming to improve opportunities to live at home as long as possible, to keep pain and discomfort at a minimum, to ensure as much time as possible with loved ones, and to enhance the person's assurance that he/she will not be abandoned by either professionals or family members. There are many variations: inpatient versus outpatient; working through community resources (e.g., Visiting Nurses Association) versus own staff; or integrated with one facility versus involvement with numerous facilities in the community. Care for the dying and for their kin and friends and anticipatory, concurrent, and postmortum grief work are going to be major tasks for collaborative endeavors of institutions, professionals, families, and other social networks (Kalish, 1985).

3. *Issues for Social Work Practice.* Social work practice is no more immune to the "disease of ageism" than are other practice professions, and it has to come to terms with it. Robert Butler defined ageism as "a process of systematic stereotyping of and discrimination against people because they are old, just as racism and sexism accomplish this with skin color and gender. Old people are categorized as senile, rigid in thought and manner, old-fashioned in morality and skills" (Butler, 1975, p. 12). Richard Kalish described another form of "ageism" that is perpetrated as much by advocates of the elderly as by their adversaries. This form of ageism equates all elderly with the least capable, least healthy, least alert, and most dependent among them. A proliferation of services is sought to improve the lot of these unfortunate people, without any awareness that these services may eventually reduce the freedom and decision-making ability of the recipients. This bias is based on two types of failure models: the "incompetence model" and the "geriactivist" model. The first is used to secure funding by pulling on the heartstrings to provide for the "incompetent" elderly, while "geriactivism" prescribes activism as the only acceptable activity for the elderly, who are charged with the obligation to stand up for their rights or be relegated to a status of "part of the problem." He proposes the "personal growth model" based on the notion that it is indeed possible and natural for elders to continue to grow (Kalish, 1979).

4. *Who Is the "Client?"* There is a tendency among social workers and other professionals to view older people primarily as recipients of services. Contrary to this view, the elderly are also an important resource. As already stated, they are a source of support to spouse, children, grandchildren, siblings, and others. At one level, the client may be the older spouse or adult child who is experiencing difficulty in the role of caregiver. At another level, the family unit may be the client, in the complex relationships and mutual reciprocity involved in giving and receiving help, or the older person may be the client either as a recipient or as a provider of services. The social worker, aware of the interdependence of family members and the role of elders as providers as well as recipients of services, will carefully address the needs of the total family network; during the process of assessing who the client is, one group may emerge as the primary client while others take a secondary place. Alternatively, the social worker may

assess multiple groups of primary clients and work with each individually or assess the family as the client and work with the family as an interacting system.

As consumers and producers of goods and services, older people constitute an economic resource and in the political arena they are active citizens. They are teachers of oral history as they communicate their life experiences; they also transmit values and traditions to subsequent generations. They act as "role models" to the young on how to mature and grow older since they are living witnesses of past events who have endured and persevered throughout the economic, political, technological, cultural, and social upheavals in this century.

Within the context of environment and specific situation, plus the unique history of each older person, each of their "needs" have to be negotiated at the later phases of life to cope with stresses of transitions, of physical and social environmental problems, and of interpersonal relationships (Lowy and O'Connor, 1986).

Coping needs come into play to meet survival concerns through adapting to conditions associated with aging processes, such as reductions in energy and bio-physiological-psychological changes, modifications in social positions and roles, in income, health, social affiliations, in interpersonal relationships, and in a sense of identity. At the same time, there is an increase in disposable time, there are different perceptions of time, of past, present, and future and, for many, an appreciable degree of freedom from certain role obligations.

Expressive needs are strivings associated with fulfilling oneself by engaging in activities for the sake of the activity itself and not necessarily to accomplish a task or reach a goal that is instrumental to something else. *Contributive needs* are predicated on the assumption that people want to give to others, such as their families, friends, peers, neighbors, and to their communities. *Influencing needs* seek to satisfy a sense of mastery; *transcendental needs* strive to overcome ego-preoccupation to move toward ego-transcendence. This task involves coming to terms with the prospect and meaning of dying and death. The need for transcendence implies a desire to become "something better" than one has been and to leave a legacy. It is a need to rise above and beyond the limitations of declining physical powers and of a diminishing life expectancy.

In addressing transcendental, coping, expressive, contributive, and influencing needs, social workers help older persons, their families, and peers in the struggle to come to terms with their existence. Social workers must be aware that elders require active outreach and are also resistant to intervention. Above all, older persons need patient listeners who know how to use "reminiscing" in the service of a person's ego (Lowy and O'Connor, 1986).

ISSUES FOR THE SOCIAL WORK PROFESSION

Specialization versus Generic Social Work

Social work with the aging makes use of specialized knowledge about aging and the aged but deploys generic methods and skills in performing social work tasks incumbent upon the practitioner in working with older persons.

In 1983, the Council on Social Work Education received a grant from the Administration on Aging to expand and strengthen the capability of social work faculties and programs to prepare practitioners and to train students at the master's and baccalaureate levels for practice with an increasingly larger aged population. The project finished its tasks in 1984 and, as a result, a network of faculty liaisons has been established in each graduate school of social work to assist in the dissemination of information and the promotion of gerontology. Many undergraduate program directors are serving in the same role.

The project has produced and disseminated four volumes dealing with the *Integration of Gerontology into Social Work Educational Curricula; Specialized Course Outlines for Gerontological Social Work Education; Curriculum Concentration in Gerontology for Graduate Social Work Education;* and *Faculty Development and Continuing Education* (Schneider and Nelson, 1985).

In 1985 another AOA grant enabled CSWE to develop "modules on aging" for undergraduate faculties and students. Training sessions for selected faculty have been held all over the country to learn to utilize these modules as quickly as possible (Greene, 1986b).

The Nature of Direct Services

What are "direct services" to the aged? Are they to be means-tested social services or social-utility services? Are they to be intensive-treatment oriented services or care-managerial services? Are they to be more supportive or more protective services? Are they personal social services or social and health care services?

Differential Use of Personpower in Providing Services

The field of aging offers many opportunities to deploy a range of personnel: professional, paraprofessional, and volunteer. Professional social workers on the M.S.W. and B.A. levels are called upon to perform many tasks in practice. Although differential competencies of trained social workers with M.S.W. and B.A. degrees have been delineated by the National Association of Social Workers, there are still many overlaps of functions between these two types, and the shortage of professional social work personnel as a result of a reluctance to work with the elderly is a major problem, especially since the demand for gerontological social workers in the next fifteen or twenty years seems great.

CONCLUSION

One of the major issues facing our graying society is in the realm of ethics. For example: the right to die with dignity, the right to initiate and withhold treatment, the appropriate allocation of national resources to an increasingly older population with a decreasing dependency ratio, the attempt to artificially prolong the life span without concern for the quality of life. Legal/medical arguments are conflicting and social work as a profession has not been very articulate in voicing its positions on such ethical issues.

Another hot issue will remain the question of ''age-integration versus age-segregation'' of programs and services. Strong arguments for age-segregated services can be made on the basis that the special problems of the elderly require the expertise of age specialists and that in times of limited resources the needs of the elderly will be neglected if they have to compete with the young. Furthermore, a number of elderly do prefer age-homogeneous interaction, especially among those considered target groups for services. Given the nature of power-brokering in our society, the elderly need a power base to be creditable in the political arena and to face competing interests from a position of strengths commensurate with their numbers and contributions in the past, present, and future, particularly during our present era of Reaganomics. Block grants pose problems for both advocates of particularism and universalism in social policy for the elderly. Elderly policy particularism has the advantage of ensuring that the elderly's unique needs will be addressed through programs tailored specifically for the elderly. It also leads to programs around which the elderly can rally and defend against budget cutters. Nonetheless, elderly policy particularism has its disadvantages as well. First, it is in part a strategy by nonpoor elderly to gain access to social services, which may result in the needs of the poor elderly being neglected even in programs specifically designed for the elderly. Second, elderly policy particularism isolates the elderly and reduces their willingness to work with other needy groups promoting more effective social policies (Neugarten, 1982).

As the strengths of young-older and old-older persons contribute toward developing a more assured self-image of the aging and toward reducing negative views and stereotypes of them by younger people, the likelihood of a more equitable partnership between young and old increases, especially if the younger generation recognizes that they too will get older in due course and some of them will wield political and economic power in a relatively short time from now. What is urgently needed is a system of linkages of age-concentrated programs and services with age-neutral programs and services based on a social policy that is informed by an inclusive view of human needs based on distributive social justice. Upon this foundation the social work profession can continue to build its micro- and macropractice in the service of the old and the young.

REFERENCES

Annual Report (1984). Massachusetts Executive Office of Elder Affairs, Commonwealth of Massachusetts.

Atchley, Robert C. (1977). *The Social Forces in Later Life*. Belmont, Calif.: Wadsworth.

Bartlett, H. (1970). *The Common Base of Social Work Practice*. New York: NASW.

Binstock, R. H. (1986). Public policy and the elderly. *Journal of Geriatric Psychiatry,* 19 (2), 115–43.

Birren, J., and Sloane, R. (Eds.) (1980). *Handbook of Mental Health and Aging.* Englewood Cliffs, N.J.: Prentice-Hall.

Brody, E. (1986). Aged in services. *Encyclopedia of Social Work.* Vol. 18, pp. 106–26. Washington, D.C.: National Association of Social Workers.

Butler, R. (1975). *Why Survive?* New York: Harper and Row.

Comfort, A. (1976). *A Good Age.* New York: Crown.

Commager, H. S. (1985). Social Security at 50. In *Modern Maturity.* Washington, D.C., 31.

Compton, B., and Galaway, B. (1975). *Social Work Process.* Homewood, Ill.: Dorset Press.

Council on Social Work Education (1958). Toward better understanding of the aging and social work education for better services to the aging. Proceedings.

Estes, C. L. (1979).*The Aging Enterprise.* San Francisco: Jossey-Bass.

Eyde, D. R., and Rich, J. (1983). *Psychological Distress in Aging: A Family Management Model.* Rockville, Md.: Aspen Publications.

Gerontological Society of America (1945–1987). Washington, D.C.

Gitterman, A. and Shulman, L. (1986). *Mutual Aid Groups and the Life Cycle.* Itasca, Ill.: Peacock Publishing.

Goldfarb, A. (1965). Psychodynamics and the three-generation family. In E. Shanas and G. Streib (Eds.), *Social Structures and the Family,* pp. 10–45. Englewood Cliffs, N.J.: Prentice-Hall.

Greene, R. A. (1986a). *Social Work with the Aging and Their Families.* New York: Aldine de Gruyter Publications.

Greene, R. A. (1986b). *Undergraduate Project of Council on Social Work Education.* Washington, D.C.: CSWE.

Hudson, R. (1981). *The Aging in Politics, Process and Policy.* Springfield, Ill.: Charles Thomas.

Huttman, E. D. (1985). *Social Services for the Elderly,* pp. 210–36. New York: The Free Press.

Journal of Gerontological Social Work (1985–1986).

Kalish, R. A. (1979). The new agism and the failure models: A polemic. *The Gerontologist,* 19 (4), 398–402.

Kalish, R. A. (1985). Services for the dying. In A. Monk (Ed.), *Handbook of Gerontological Services,* pp. 531–46. New York: Van Nostrand Reinhold.

Kennedy, J. F. (1963). Address to Congress. The elderly citizens of our nation. *Congressional Record.* Washington, D.C.: U.S. Government Printing Office.

Kubie, S., and Landau, G. (1953). *Group Work with the Aged.* New York: International University Press.

Lowenthal, M. F., Chiroboza, D., and Thurnber, M. (1975). *The Four Stages of Life.* San Francisco: Jossey-Bass.

Lowy, L. (1974). *The Function of Social Work in a Changing Society..* Boston: Charles River Books.

Lowy, L. (1982, November). Social Security intergenerational problem. *The World,* pp. 3–4. Boston: University News.

Lowy, L. (1985). *Social Work with the Aging.* 2d ed. New York: Longman Publishers, Inc.

Lowy, L., and O'Connor, D. (1986). *Education in the Later Years.* Lexington, Mass.: Lexington Books.

McClusky, H. Y., and the Technical Committee on Education (1971). *Background and Issues—Report for the 1971 White House Conference on Aging.* Washington, D.C.: U.S. Government Printing Office.

Mace, N. L., and Rabins, P. U. (1982). *The Thirty-Six Hour Day: A Family Guide to Caring for Persons with Alzheimer's Disease, Related Dementing Illness and Memory Loss in Later Life.* Baltimore: Johns Hopkins University Press.

McMaldonado, D., Jr. (1986). Aged. *Encyclopedia of Social Work.* Vol. 18, pp. 95–106. Washington, D.C.: National Association of Social Workers.

Meyer, C. H. (Ed.) (1986). *Social Work with the Aging.* 2d ed. Washington, D.C.: National Association of Social Workers.

Monk, A. (1981). Social work with the aged: Principles of practice. *Social Work, 26,* 61–88.

Monk, A. (Ed.) (1985). *Handbook of Gerontological Services.* New York: Van Nostrand Reinhold.

National Conference of Social Workers Proceedings (1947). Washington, D.C.: National Association of Social Workers.

Nelson, G. M., and Schneider, R. L. (1984). The current status of gerontology. *Graduate Social Work Education.* Washington, D.C.: CSWE Series in Gerontology.

Neugarten, B. L. (1982). *Age or Need? Public Policies for Older People.* Beverly Hills, Calif.: Sage.

Older Americans Act of 1965, as amended; P. L. 95–178. Administration of Aging. Washington, D.C.: DHHS, 1987.

Pincus, A. and Monahan, A. (1972). *Social Work Practice.* Itasca, Ill.: F. E. Peacock.

Rathbone-McCuan, E., and Coward, R. T. (1985). Respite and adult day care services. In A. Monk (Ed.), *Handbook of Gerontological Services,* pp. 457–82. New York: Van Nostrand Reinhold.

Rubinow, I. M. (1930). The care of the aged. Proceedings of the Deutsch Foundation Conference.

Schneider, R. and Nelson, G. (1985). *The National Curriculum Project in Gerontology.* New York: CSWE.

Schottland, C. I. (1970). *The Social Security Program in the United States.* (Unpublished manuscript.)

Schulz, J. (1985). *The Economics of Aging.* 3d ed. Belmont, Calif.: Wadsworth.

Shulman, L. (1986). *The Skills of Helping Individuals and Groups.* Itaska, Ill.: F. E. Peacock Pub.

Silverstone, B., and Burack-Weiss, A. (1983). *Social Work Practice with the Frail Elderly and Their Families: The Auxiliary Function Model.* Springfield, Ill.: Charles C. Thomas.

Siporin, M. (1975). *Introduction to Social Work Practice.* New York: Macmillan.

Social Casework (1954). 35 (7), 299–300.

Social Security Act, Title II, Social Insurance, U.S. Code starting at 42 USC 401- Title XVIII (Medicare), Title XIX (Medicaid), Title XX (Social Services).

Social Service Review (1952). 26 (2), 181–94.

Social Work Yearbook (1949). New York: Russell Sage Foundation.

The State of Families 1984–85 (1985). Report by the Family Service America, New York.

Steinberg, R. M., and Carter, G. W. (1983). *Casemanagement and the Elderly*. Lexington, Mass.: Lexington Books.

U.S. General Accounting Office (1987). Report by the Comptroller General. Washington, D.C.: GAO.

White House Conference on Aging, 1961 (1962). The nation and its older people. Washington, D.C.: U.S. Government Printing Office.

White House Conference on Aging, 1971 (1971). Toward a national policy on aging. Vols. 1 and 2. Washington, D.C.: U.S. Government Printing Office.

Wickenden, E. (1953). *The Needs of Older People and Public Welfare Services to Meet Them*. Chicago: American Public Welfare Association.

9. AFTERWORD. FACING THE FRONTIERS: INTERDISCIPLINARY ISSUES AND AGENDAS

Joan B. Wood, Iris A. Parham, and Jodi L. Teitelman

On the frontier for educational gerontology lie the complex and challenging issues relating to professionalization of the field. At present, there are no national standards for structure or content of academic programs in gerontology. Nor are there guidelines for gerontology instruction. Gerontologists do not agree among themselves as to whether gerontology is a discipline, a multidisciplinary area of study, or a profession. Will gerontology become an academically established discipline with its own degree-awarding departments? Or will it become subsumed under the auspices of other disciplines as an area of specialization?

Gerontology credentials of various denominations including degrees and certificates at graduate and undergraduate levels are currently awarded by numerous academic institutions. There is little agreement about the meaning or value of these various credentials.

Nor is there agreement as to the appropriate relationship between geriatrics and gerontology. Is one a science and the other a field of practice? Or does each combine elements of both science and practice? Do gerontology and geriatrics share a common multidisciplinary core of knowledge from which both can benefit?

What role will accreditation play in the future of academic gerontology? Is licensure of practitioners foreseeable in the future?

These issues are important to students planning for careers in aging, to young professionals struggling to establish their identities, and to educational administrators weighing the allocation of resources. The Association for Gerontology in Higher Education (AGHE) and other professional organizations will likely be in the forefront as gerontologists attempt to grapple with these issues.

In 1984 AGHE established a standards committee, and several studies are currently being conducted to provide a data base from which to develop gerontology curriculum standards. Data on the current requirements of academic gerontology programs by level of education and type of credential (Peterson et al., 1987) and on faculty preparation and responsibilities have been reported (Bolton, 1988; Peterson et al., 1987). Human resource studies are also being pursued to collect data on current gerontology students, graduates of academic gerontology programs, and employers of graduates. Graduates' memberships in professional associations will also be assessed.

From the data bases provided by these studies, subcommittees of the AGHE Standards Committee will develop guidelines for gerontological education by level of education and type of credential. These guidelines will be reviewed by the full standards committee and by the AGHE Standards Task Force, composed of liaison persons appointed by national professional associations in aging to coordinate the AGHE effort with similar activities in their respective organizations. The AGHE Presidents' Commission on Standards, composed of AGHE past presidents plus the current president and president-elect, will approve both the process through which standards are developed and the standards themselves.

Throughout the standards development process, AGHE members and others in the field of gerontology will have several opportunities to contribute and to comment upon the process. The AGHE Standards Committee is an open committee with a commitment to soliciting involvement and input from all interested parties. Special sessions dealing with the standards process have been and are being held at annual conferences of AGHE, the Gerontological Society of America (GSA) (formerly the Gerontological Society), and the American Society of Aging (ASA) (formerly the Western Gerontological Society). Additionally, standards committee members are being urged to make presentations regarding the standards development process at national meetings of various disciplinary organizations, e.g., American Sociological Association, American Psychological Association (APA), National Council on Social Work Education.

The findings of the AGHE Standards Committee project are expected to be approved by the organization in early 1989. The seriousness with which this process is being pursued by gerontology educators was reflected in the size and response of the audience when the project was discussed at the annual scientific meeting of the GSA in Washington, D.C., in November 1987. A large and very vocal audience of gerontologists debated vigorously the issues raised by the effort to develop gerontological education standards (*Aging Research and Training News*, November 23, 1987).

These issues are frequently discussed by the memberships of GSA, AGHE, ASA, and the National Council on the Aging (NCOA). A brief look at the history of gerontological education in this country shows that the interdisciplinary issues and agendas on educational gerontology's frontier have also been the issues of the past. The field has evolved to a point where the need for resolution of some of these issues has arrived.

THE BEGINNINGS OF EDUCATIONAL GERONTOLOGY

In the first issue of the *Journal of Gerontology,* Lawrence K. Frank (1946) wrote that the "new" problems related to the aging of the American population "transcend the knowledge and methods of any one discipline or profession" (p. 1) and demand that the findings of many separate investigators be synthesized into a coherent whole. The Gerontological Society, which published the new journal, had been formed in 1945 to promote professional contact among scientists from a variety of disciplines who were studying aging and/or the aged (Adler, 1958). A few courses in aging were being offered around the country at that time, primarily as electives within the disciplines of biology, psychology, and sociology (American Psychological Association, 1948). A small but growing number of investigators were conducting empirical research in these areas.

A major concern in the early years related to increasing the number of college and university teachers adequately prepared to provide training in gerontology. The Gerontological Society took a leadership role in 1955 by appointing a special committee to develop plans for meeting this pressing need. Under the active direction of this committee, whose original members were James Birren, Clark Tibbitts, and Wilma Donahue, the historical course of educational gerontology was shaped. Several university training seminars and summer institutes were held. Special Ph.D. training programs with specializations in aging were developed at Washington University and the University of Chicago. Supported by grants from the National Institute of Mental Health and the National Heart Institute, an Inter-University Training Institute in Social Gerontology was established at the University of Michigan in 1957 (Donahue, 1960).

The goals of this institute were: (1) to develop what was considered to be a new scientific field, social gerontology, by collecting and systematizing existing scientific knowledge of aging; (2) to introduce this knowledge to the academic and scientific communities; and (3) to increase the number of scientists trained to teach, conduct research, and provide services in the field (Donahue, 1960). Existing scientific knowledge of aging was collected and organized into the first three handbooks of aging for dissemination as reference works in the teaching of gerontology (Birren, 1959; Burgess, 1960; Tibbitts, 1960). Five course syllabi were prepared and disseminated to aid in filling the void in instructional materials (University of Michigan Institute for Social Gerontology, 1959). Seventy-five faculty personnel representing thirty-six states and Puerto Rico were trained in two summer institutes in social gerontology in 1958 and 1959 (Donahue, 1960). These gerontology fellows constituted the cadre of instructors who were instrumental in further development of the field.

A survey of university instruction in social gerontology conducted in 1957–1958 showed that fifty institutions were offering course work or seminars in gerontology (Donahue, 1960). Research in aging was being conducted at seventy-two institutions, despite the fact that funding for other than biological research was almost nonexistent. Clearly, gerontology education had begun.

The 1961 White House Conference on Aging represented a demarcation point. At the request of leaders in the field of academic gerontology, supported by the 1961 White House Conference, the U.S. Office on Aging prepared a suggested curriculum for university programs in gerontology (U.S. Department of Health, Education and Welfare, Office on Aging, 1965).

THE GROWTH PERIOD

The 1960s and 1970s witnessed a dramatic increase in the number and diversity of gerontology education programs. Unlike the academic interest in women's studies and African studies, which flourished and waned in the context of social movements, the growth of gerontology education has been driven by demographics. Concurrent with increasing public awareness of the "graying of America" and increased demand for aging services, the number of gerontology programs in institutions of higher education increased from fewer than a dozen in the 1950s to more than 200 by the late 1970s (Craig, 1982; Johnson et al., 1980). A survey conducted by AGHE in 1976 identified more than 1,200 institutions which were offering some instruction in aging (Sprouse, 1976). Of these, 48 percent (607 institutions) offered credit courses in gerontology (Bolton et al., 1978).

A variety of program models developed as faculty and administration sought to deal with institutional contingencies in local situations. Special emphases, minors, or specializations were set up within traditional disciplinary programs (e.g., psychology, sociology, social work). Certificate programs in aging studies were established. These were sometimes offered within an existing administrative unit, but were more typically granted by a multidisciplinary center or institute established to provide university-wide coordination of studies in aging. Special programs or departments were established in some institutions to award degrees in gerontology. At the University of Southern California, a school of gerontology was established. Interestingly, all of these models developed at both undergraduate and graduate levels.

A major factor in the growth of new programs in the 1960s and 1970s was the intervention of the federal government, which began to provide funding for career preparation in aging under several initiatives. Early funding, primarily from the National Institute of Mental Health and the National Institute of Child Health and Human Development, focused on preparing professionals for careers in teaching and research (Education and Training in Gerontology—1970, 1970). The career training grant program, begun by the United States Administration on Aging (AOA) in 1966–1967, was designed to prepare practitioners for jobs in aging services programs created under the Older Americans Act. In 1976–1977, the first multidisciplinary gerontology centers were funded by the Administration on Aging to serve as centers for implementing integrated multidisciplinary programs of education, training, research, and consultation in aging.

The development of the multidisciplinary gerontology centers was a significant step in the advancement of gerontology in higher education (Simson and Wilson, 1981). With their funding, both the number and variety of academic programs in aging were substantially increased. The enabling legislation reflected a recognition at the federal level of the need to draw on the resources of various departments, schools, and facilities within an institution in order to provide a multidisciplinary approach to educational activities in aging (Administration on Aging, 1976). The need for coordination and integration of multidisciplinary efforts was stressed.

Paralleling the growth of educational programs in gerontology was the formation and development of professional organizations that engaged in activities supportive of the field. The American Psychological Association (APA) created a Division of Maturity and Old Age in 1946. A report was prepared by this division's Committee on Instruction for Maturity and Old Age, describing results of a national survey of courses in the psychology of aging (APA, 1948). The report's findings prodded the Section on Psychology and Social Sciences of the Gerontological Society to appoint the ad hoc committee of Birren, Tibbitts, and Donahue (referred to earlier), which assumed early leadership in promoting the development of university instruction in gerontology. This Gerontological Society Committee was recognized by the APA Division of Maturity and Old Age and was subsequently expanded to include representation of APA membership. The first gerontology training programs supported by the federal government were based on models that had been developed by members of the Gerontological Society and the APA Division of Maturity and Old Age (Craig, 1982).

Several other professional organizations also assumed leadership roles in attempting to establish guidelines for preparing professionals in their respective disciplines to work in the field of aging. Early examples of these include the Council on Social Work Education (1964), the Association of Collegiate Schools of Architecture (Byerts and Taylor, 1977), and the American Personnel and Guidance Association (Ganikos, 1979).

Another Gerontological Society project in 1964–1966 developed guidelines for planning and organizing graduate level programs in social gerontology (Kushner and Bunch, 1967). A decade later the Western Gerontological Society (WGS) drafted standards and guidelines for educational programs in gerontology at the associate, baccalaureate, and graduate levels (Ridley et al., 1978). Interestingly, Ridley et al. (1978) published their standards and guidelines as a "draft." This apparently reflected the authors' hesitancy in making a definitive statement, in light of the contradictory views of many aging educators with regards to the concept of gerontology as a discipline.

These positions were explored at some length in Kushner and Bunch (1967) by contributors to the volume who argued that gerontology should be considered a new interdisciplinary science or, conversely, that the study of aging should become no more than a specialized content area within established disciplines. At this juncture, the debate between those viewing gerontology as a separate discipline and those considering it to be a specialty area became a salient one.

A strong proponent of the "gerontology as discipline" view during these years was Robert Kleemeir (Kleemeir, 1965). Kleemeir, Robert Havighurst, and Clark Tibbitts wrote, in Kushner and Bunch (1967), that gerontology as "a distinctive area of research and teaching" could appropriately "be accommodated in the university structure with its own faculty, administrative authority, and academic rights and responsibilities" (Kleemeir, Havighurst, and Tibbitts, 1967). Indeed, the first master's degree programs in gerontology were established in 1967 at the University of South Florida and North Texas State University with funding from the United States Administration on Aging. Within a decade, nine additional master's degree programs had been established. A major factor in the development of these programs, as noted earlier, was the availability of career training grants from the Administration on Aging (AOA). AOA encouraged the development of autonomous professionally oriented programs. The curriculum guide developed by the Office on Aging (under Clark Tibbitts' leadership as director of research and training) following the 1961 White House Conference on Aging suggested content and administrative organization for a two-year interdisciplinary graduate program, adaptable for training both generalists and professional personnel (U.S. Department of HEW, Office on Aging, 1965). It is likely that many institutions opted to create a degree program rather than a specialization within an established department as a means of enhancing their chances for funding (Peterson and Bolton, 1980).

Throughout the 1970s, as the numbers of academic gerontology programs increased, the issue of what gerontology was and should be was debated (Peterson and Bolton, 1980; Seltzer, Sterns, and Hickey, 1978; Sterns et al., 1979). In 1978, during a national colloquium on higher education and aging, Tibbitts predicted "formal acceptance of gerontology as a scientific discipline" (p. 14) within the relatively near future (Tibbitts, 1980). According to Tibbitts, institutes, schools, and departments of gerontology would appear in greater numbers to accommodate "a conceptual structure and expanding body of tested knowledge already so vast as to require specialization within the field" (p. 14). Conversely, in the introduction to the proceedings of this invitational colloquium, Harold R. Johnson (1980) wrote that gerontology lacked the knowledge base, the professional skills, and the research methods to qualify as either a discipline or a profession and did not "deserve to be viewed as either" (p. 4). He was willing to grant that, within the foreseeable future, gerontology would emerge as a profession or as a specialization within professions, but not as a discipline. In this environment of strong, opposing opinions about the future of academic gerontology, the Foundations Project (Johnson et al., 1980) was conceived.

THE SELF-SCRUTINY PHASE

With the rapid proliferation of gerontology instruction in higher education, early concerns for creating and developing programs were replaced by concerns about the quality of those programs. Professional organizations and federal funding agencies, which played important roles in the growth and development of educational gerontology, were also instrumental in this phase of self-assessment. A joint research project of the Association for Gerontology in Higher Education (AGHE) and the Gerontological Society (GS), entitled "Foundations for Establishing Educational Program Standards in Gerontology," was funded by the Administration on Aging in 1978.

The principal goals of this project were: (1) to determine whether a consensus of opinion existed regarding a core of knowledge in the field of aging, (2) to identify the topical components of educational programs in gerontology, and (3) to produce basic guidelines for curriculum development (Johnson et al., 1980). The project committee recognized the necessity of resolving many issues in gerontological education before the issue of program standards could be dealt with. Central to this dilemma was the controversy within academic gerontology about the nature and status of the field.

The data reported from a national survey revealed a clear consensus among experts in the field of aging that a core knowledge base in gerontology exists, suggesting gerontology to be a distinct field of study. The project committee concluded, however, that the existence of a knowledge base did not indicate whether gerontology should be developed as a distinct discipline, as a multidisciplinary area, or as a profession (Johnson et al., 1980). They did agree that the core curriculum was multidisciplinary in nature and concluded that the establishment of educational program standards in gerontology would be premature at that time.

The findings of the Foundations Project did not resolve the issues of gerontology's future, but rather signaled the beginning of a period of serious self-scrutiny. Several environmental factors had an impact on this continued introspection in the field of aging. One important influence was the decline in federal funding for career training projects.

An AOA-funded Gerontology Education Data Project at the University of Nebraska in 1977 found that over one-third of all financial support for gerontology education programs was provided by the federal government (Bolton et al., 1978). More than half the institutional programs begun before 1980 had been initiated with federal funding (Craig, 1982; Peterson, 1987). Reduction in federal funds allocated for academic gerontology programs in the early 1980s and plans by federal officials to terminate such support spurred the development of projects to assess the impact of these actions. Efforts to seek other sources of funding (e.g., foundations, institutional) and the resulting need to justify their existence also forced programs to reevaluate their goals and purposes, to assess the appropriateness of training delivered in relation to job market demands, and to seek strategies for achieving organizational stability (Craig, 1982; Hartford, 1980; Mangum and Rich, 1980; Seltzer, 1982).

Professional organizations assisted in efforts to assess the growth of programs and plan for human resource needs in specific disciplines (APA, 1985; Myers, 1983; Nelson and Schneider, 1984). For example, a national conference on training psychologists for work in aging in the challenging environment of the 1980s was held in Boulder, Colorado, in 1981 (Santos and VandenBos, 1982).

At least one statewide effort was made to assess the status of gerontology in higher education. A statewide task force of gerontology educators and service providers, which was convened by the Virginia Center on Aging at Virginia Commonwealth University, the State Council on Higher Education, and the Virginia Office on Aging, prepared a report on gerontology programs at colleges and universities in Virginia (Arling and Romaniuk, 1980). The task force identified various work roles in different job classifications in the field of aging, delineated the knowledge and skills needed to meet these work roles, and constructed content objectives for educational programs to prepare workers for these roles.

In the course of these evaluative efforts, a number of "disciplinary" issues were raised. The first of these had to do with whether the core content areas identified in the Foundations Project were included in existing programs. Van Orman (1984) found that 66 percent of the undergraduate programs listed in the 1982 AGHE *National Directory of Educational Programs in Gerontology* (Sullivan, 1982) included at least two-thirds of the forty-five content areas. Peterson (1984) found that master's degree programs in gerontology were very similar in content and generally consistent with the content areas recommended by the Foundations Project. Peterson (1984) also found that the programs were well within the standards set by the Council of Graduate Schools and the guidelines established by the Education Committee of the Western Gerontological Society (Ridley et al., 1978). Peterson concluded that the programs could legitimately be viewed as comparable preparation for employment in the field of aging and, as such, could be considered a base for beginning discussions concerning professional accreditation.

Peterson and Bolton (1980) believed, as did Levine (1981), that gerontology did not meet the criteria for a discipline (Dressel and Mayhew, 1974). Spence (1983) shared this view, but argued that many of the problems experienced by existing gerontology programs had arisen because of lack of a strong administrative power base. He believed that autonomous programs offered through formally sanctioned structures, such as departments of gerontology with independent budgets, would be essential for survival in higher education.

Peterson (1978) provided the most comprehensive analysis of the issue of structure in the longevity of educational gerontology programs. Utilizing four factors (curricula, faculty, administration, and students), he considered the various types of existing organizational arrangements. Peterson concluded that the structure of a gerontology program is a primary reflection of the extent to which faculty are able to control the program. Faculty control over all aspects of the program is more readily provided in autonomous administrative units, such as departments or schools. It is important to note the impact of faculty control on the development and continuation of gerontology programs in academia.

A randomly sampled survey of the memberships of the Gerontological Society of America (GSA) and the Western Gerontological Society (WGS) indicated gerontology's development as a professional field (Hirschfield and Peterson, 1982). This was seen both in perceptions of the GSA and WGS memberships and in terms of meeting criteria for a profession. Criteria being met, as indicated by data from the survey, include: (1) full-time occupational participation in the field, (2) formal degree programs based on a specialized body of knowledge, (3) academic journals disseminating knowledge, and (4) professional organizations which speak for the field. Professional criteria not being met were: (1) restricted membership in professional societies, (2) a code of ethics, (3) standards for accreditation of academic programs, and (4) a process for licensure.

Many of those who argued in recent years that gerontology was not a discipline based their positions on perceptions of limitations in the development of a body of theory and lack of a methodology specific to the study of aging (Peterson, 1987). Seltzer (1983, 1985), who has been the most eloquent spokesperson for viewing gerontology as a discipline in the 1980s, asserted that gerontology is developing its own language, concepts, and methods which may not always be "necessarily original to itself, yet the blending of elements from more traditional fields may result in a new whole, qualitatively different from the sum of its parts" (Seltzer, 1983, p. 4). Atchley (1985) pointed out that most of the numerous theories of social gerontology are relatively unknown in the other social sciences. Using the same rationale as Seltzer (1983, 1985) and Atchley (1985), Bramwell (1985) also argued that gerontology should be considered as a discipline. "Disciplines arise or are invented: they are not discovered," Bramwell (1985, p. 209) pointed out. Gerontology is evolving in much the same way that psychology, social work, and other disciplines developed some years ago.

Seltzer (1983, 1985) suggested that the time had arrived in the developmental history of academic gerontology for gerontologists to redirect their energies from self-conscious, introspective activities to issues of criteria for accreditation of programs and credentialing of practitioners. The AGHE Project on Enhancing the Quality of Gerontology Instruction, commonly referred to as the AGHE-USC survey (Peterson et al., 1987), was seen as the first step in providing data to guide future development of the field. This survey provided a data base on the extent and character of gerontology instruction in higher education, to be used by the AGHE Standards Committee in preparing guidelines for program development. The vocal and vigorous expression of differing opinions concerning the standards process, as discussed at national conferences in 1987 and 1988, indicates that many members of professional gerontological organizations do not share Seltzer's vision of the future of academic gerontology.

THE PROFESSIONALIZATION OF GERONTOLOGY

Programs of gerontology instruction in institutions of higher education have increased dramatically over the past thirty years (Peterson et al., 1987). The 1987 AGHE-USC survey identified 1,155 campuses on which at least one gerontology course was regularly taught for credit. More than 700 programs of instruction in gerontology (defined as a minimum of four gerontology courses) were identified on 351 campuses. A total of 408 programs culminated in the awarding of a gerontology credential (e.g., certificate, degree, minor, major, concentration).

The results of the AGHE-USC survey (Peterson et al., 1987) indicated that the number of campuses offering gerontology credit courses had almost doubled since the 1977 Nebraska study (Bolton et al., 1978). Peterson et al. (1987) found that most courses had been started within the previous ten years, with 25 percent having begun since 1980. These findings were particularly encouraging in view of the changes in federal funding for gerontology education and training programs in recent years.

Data from the AGHE-USC survey indicate that federal funding is currently not a major source of gerontology program support (Peterson et al., 1987). Federal funds, where available, are very limited, and funding periods are abbreviated. Few institutions rely on federal grants to support gerontology programs. While federal funds were undoubtedly a significant factor during the early years of program development, most programs of gerontology instruction in higher education were initiated without federal dollars. Peterson et al. (1987) found that over 73 percent of program support for gerontology had come from institutional sources, with the highest level of federal support (15.3 percent) reported by programs begun before 1971.

Craig (1982) posited that maturity of gerontology programs could best be measured by their stability, particularly in the absence of continued federal support. The AGHE-USC survey indicated: (1) that other resources for funding gerontology instruction have been tapped, (2) that many gerontology programs have achieved both financial and organizational stability, and (3) that instructional programs in gerontology continue to increase in number.

These developments, and recent attention given to these concerns in professional organizations (e.g., AGHE Standards Committee) and in the academic literature (Hirschfield and Peterson, 1982; Peterson, 1984, 1987; Seltzer, 1983, 1985), portend consideration of a number of issues related to professionalization of the field. Among these are accreditation of educational programs in gerontology and credentialing or licensure of professionals in the field of aging. Despite vehement opposition among many gerontologists to both accreditation and licensure, extant data indicate that gerontology is moving toward becoming both an academic discipline and a profession. Examination of the criteria for an academic discipline, even by those who contend that gerontology is not likely to become a discipline within the near future, indicates that gerontology has developed or is developing many of them (Bramwell, 1985; Johnson, 1980; Peterson and Bolton, 1980; Levine, 1981; Seltzer, 1985).

A crucial issue in the discussion of the status of gerontology as discipline is the purpose of academic gerontology. Peterson (1987) views gerontology as service-oriented, with a primary concern for development of knowledge and skills to train workers in the field of aging. Seltzer (1983), in contrast, sees the primary purpose of academic gerontology as identical to that of other disciplines, i.e., the creation and communication of a body of knowledge for its own sake. Peterson (1987) acknowledges that simply because gerontology does not at present meet the criteria of a discipline does not mean that it will never do so. Inevitably, regardless of current controversy, the issue of accreditation is on gerontology's frontier.

Accreditation is the process of evaluating the quality of an educational program for the purpose of determining whether acceptable standards for such a program have been or are being met. The process of accreditation presupposes the existence of standards. Seltzer (1985) addressed both the pros and cons of accreditation for academic gerontology programs. Reasons for accreditation include: (1) to provide students with information about the credibility of various programs for use in making choices about where to matriculate; (2) to protect the public and the profession of gerontology from the phenomenon of the "instant gerontologist," i.e., individuals promoting themselves as experts in aging without appropriate training or credentials; and (3) to provide educational administrators with information about faculty competencies and curriculum adequacies in a new discipline (Seltzer, 1985).

A number of potentially problematic issues must be dealt with in establishing an accreditation process. These include such questions as what is to be accredited, how the process will take place, who will do the accrediting, and what criteria will be used for accreditation. Will these include standards for faculty competence and administrative structure as well as for courses and course content? Will there be criteria for determining the competencies of graduates? Will the criteria established be minimum standards for acceptability or will they be standards of excellence? Seltzer (1985) foresees problems if political and administrative issues become embroiled in the accreditation process. The process itself must be delineated, decisions about the accrediting organization must be made, and issues of expense and time must be considered.

Peterson (1984) suggested that the similarity in content and approach to professional training in master's degree programs in gerontology across the United States warrants consideration of accreditation. Seltzer (1983, 1985) called for a "Criteria Project" that would build on materials developed by the Western Gerontological Society (Ridley et al., 1978) and the AGHE-GSA Foundations Project (Johnson et al., 1980) to begin developing standards and procedures for the accreditation of academic gerontology programs. The AGHE Standards Project was not directly initiated in response to Peterson, Seltzer, and others with similar views. Rather, the project was begun in response to continuing requests from educational institutions over several years for information about how to establish gerontology programs. (To further meet this need, AGHE has also published a series of brief bibliographies on various content areas to serve as a resource for faculty and administrators seeking to develop gerontological instruction programs.)

The AGHE Standards Project was completed in early 1989. Whether the work of this project will become the basis for an accreditation process in academic gerontology is impossible to foresee. Perhaps gerontologists will continue to follow the philosophy expressed by Storandt (1978) in seeking to socialize rather than legislate the quality of gerontology programs. The issue of acceptable standards for gerontology programs in higher education is far from settled.

A related but more complex issue involves the credentialing of professional gerontological practitioners. Hirschfield and Peterson (1982) demonstrated that gerontology is progressing along the continuum of development as a profession. Estimations of the extent to which gerontology has developed as a profession depend upon "which model one uses" (Hirschfield and Peterson, 1982, p. 217). This issue may seem somewhat less controversial in the current gerontology literature only because it is less often discussed. Certainly, the issue of licensing gerontologists will not be uncontroversial.

Many practitioners in the field of aging continue to define their practice in terms of their original profession (e.g., social work, sociology, medicine, psychology) and consider gerontology or geriatrics to be subspecialties. Psychologists at the Older Boulder Conference in 1981 recommended that licensure standards continue to be defined in terms of practice in "the major field of psychology (e.g., clinical)" rather than in geropsychology, which was viewed as a smaller subspecialty or interest area (Niederehe, 1982, p. 139). There is no indication that consideration was given to credentialing gerontologists as a separate profession.

Credentialing and licensing are, as is accreditation, legitimating processes. The major distinction is that accreditation legitimates an educational program or institution, while credentialing and licensure are designed to assess the competency of individuals. There are many who will argue that professional practitioners in the field of aging are adequately credentialed by the degrees, diplomas, or certificates awarded to them upon successful completion of programs of study in gerontology. They may be further legitimated by membership in professional organizations in gerontology, although such membership is not restricted beyond the requirement of some organizations for sponsorship by a current member. Those who favor certification or licensing will note that many educational programs do not award a credential and that there is little consistency in requirements among those which do (Peterson et al., 1987). Further, many faculty have themselves become credentialed by research and publications in the field of aging rather than by formal training (Bolton, 1988).

The major argument advanced in favor of licensing is quality control, i.e., the need to protect consumers of services and the public in general from "instant gerontologists" who, in their ignorance, continue to spread myths and stereotypes about aging and the aged (Seltzer, 1985). Second, it is presumed that regulation not only protects the public but also ensures that services are continuously improved (Hogan, 1979). Licensure should, therefore, result in improved standards for both education and service in aging. A third argument is that licensing gerontological practitioners may make them eligible for third-party payments. Conversely, untrained persons could be barred from licensing and, thereby, from third-party reimbursement (Seltzer, 1985).

The arguments against licensure of gerontologists are also many. Seltzer (1985) points out that when licensing is implemented in a new field, existing practitioners who may not meet licensing requirements are typically ''grandparented'' into the licensed practitioner community. Such a practice would do little to alleviate the current problem of lack of competence in aging existing among some service providers. A related concern is that licensing requirements are often based on entry-level skills, or minimum levels of competency, and seldom address issues of incompetent practice unless dramatic evidence of fraudulent, unethical, or criminal behavior is presented (Danish and Smyer, 1981; Seltzer, 1985).

Another argument against licensing relates to the benefits ostensibly derived by consumers from regulation of professional activities in this manner. Licensing tends to restrict the number of practitioners in a given field, usually resulting in higher prices to the consumer and decreased utilization of services. Licensed practitioners tend to move into private practice (Danish and Smyer, 1981). This could potentially result in a dangerous disruption of aging services delivery, since many services for older adults are currently available only in the public sector. Licensing could also create antagonism among professional gerontologists. Danish (1980) described conflicts that have arisen at many levels within the field of psychology as a result of licensing.

Licensing boards typically consist of political appointees with little consumer representation (Danish and Smyer, 1981; Seltzer, 1985). Consequently, conflicts of interest may be created as control of licensing boards remains in the hands of those the boards seek to regulate. Professional self-regulation is not necessarily harmful if, in practice, it protects the public or facilitates human interaction so as to meet the needs of the public (Hogan, 1979). Viewed from this perspective, licensing may function more in the best interests of practitioners than in those of consumers (Danish and Smyer, 1981; Gross, 1978; Matarazzo, 1977; Seltzer, 1985).

Indeed, the most serious indictment of licensure is the unintended effects on the consumer of services (Danish and Smyer, 1981). Licensing of service providers is frequently based on the medical model, which has significant implications for the self-image and self-concept of individuals seeking services (Danish and Smyer, 1981; Seltzer, 1985). In this model, clients are ''patients'' or ''people with a problem'' who, by virtue of the circumstances of service delivery, see themselves as incapable of helping themselves and thus are relieved of the responsibility to do so. The professional practitioner is seen as a specialist who is able to solve the problems of others. Family and friends who comprise social support systems may also feel relieved of responsibility for the problem and may actually withdraw support that might otherwise be offered (Danish and Smyer, 1981). Consequently, problems that may arise from social inequities are often treated as though they are individual in origin (Seltzer, 1985).

The stages in the evolution of a profession, identified by Hirschfield and Peterson (1982) and by Matarazzo (1977), indicate that the logical progression following the accreditation of academic programs is the certification or licensure of graduates. As Seltzer (1985) has pointed out, timing is a critical issue, i.e., is the time right for licensure of gerontologists? A general review of licensure problems in related fields seems to indicate that licensing may not adequately address current concerns regarding protection of the elderly consumer and quality control of service delivery by the profession. Perhaps those issues can be better dealt with in alternate ways. Efforts can be made to incorporate requirements for gerontology training into qualifications for jobs in the field of aging (Seltzer, 1985). Professional organizations and educational institutions can begin to address and define the issues of competency-based education, especially in field work or internships. Certification of practitioners, which would limit use of the title "gerontologist" to those who have met specified qualifications, may be pursued as an alternative to licensure. Assessment center methodology that provides detailed assessment of skills demonstrated in standardized performance situations (Koocher, 1979) could be utilized in granting certification.

Many academic gerontologists consider other issues to be more immediate. Such issues include: (1) defining the job market and preparing graduates for it, (2) the feasibility and marketability of either dual degrees or a Ph.D. in gerontology, and (3) the as-yet-unresolved relationship between gerontology and geriatrics. A central concern among gerontology educators in an environment of declining resources for human services is the availability of jobs for graduates. Two national surveys of graduate gerontology degree programs have found that approximately 60 percent of those responding were employed in the field of aging (Ketron, Inc., 1981; Peterson, 1985). Those individuals who had had work experience in aging before entering the degree program were more likely to have secured employment in aging than those who had no such previous work history (Ketron, Inc., 1981; Peterson, 1985). Skeptics have pointed to this as evidence that previous work history rather than a degree in gerontology is the key factor in employment experiences of graduates (Krause, 1987). In any event, much attention has been focused on human resource studies in projections for various job markets in the field of aging (Peterson, 1987; Williams, 1987).

One frequently discussed option for enhancing graduates' opportunities in the job market is awarding dual degrees in gerontology and more traditional, related disciplines (e.g., psychology, social work, sociology). Forty-six percent of a representative sampling of the Western Gerontological Society membership and 35 percent of a representative sample of Gerontological Society of America members favored dual degrees for students interested in working with older adults (Hirschfield and Peterson, 1982).

Presumably, the educational impact of a dual degree would result in a more competent professional. Experience from other dual degree programs has indicated that these programs are appealing to modern students who are concerned with maximizing their attractiveness in the job market (Rich et al., 1986). Duplication of course content should be reduced from current models (e.g., specializations, certificates) and a combined practicum experience could be designed to meet requirements of both programs. However, dual degree programs incorporating gerontology have remained few in number. Administrative concerns related to development and management of such programs (e.g., the complications inherent in curriculum adaptations and the double counting of courses, administrative requirements of faculty which would reduce time for teaching and research) have probably been a factor in this situation (Rich et al., 1986).

Increased societal demands for professionals with special skills in aging (Kahl, 1976; Kane et al., 1980; National Association of Social Workers, 1983; National Institute on Aging, 1984) coupled with the increasing professionalization of gerontology have led several American universities to contemplate instituting doctoral programs in gerontology. Ph.D. programs in gerontology with a specialization in social policy are being planned at the University of Southern California and the University of Massachusetts. Preliminary discussions relative to Ph.D. programs in gerontology are in progress at the University of South Florida and Virginia Commonwealth University.

The rationale for these programs is based on the level of development of gerontology as an academic and professional field which necessitates graduates' specialization. Approximately seventy university programs already offer courses or concentrations in aging at the doctoral level (APA, 1985; Lobenstine, 1985). Further specialization in the field is limited by the rarity of independent programs at the Ph.D. level. These programs would more effectively foster a high level of scholarship in aging than the current practice of specializing or concentrating in aging within traditional academic departments. Students would approach questions from the integrated perspective of gerontology rather than from the standpoint of another discipline. Development and implementation of doctoral level programs would move gerontology further along the continuum of professionalization. Thus, it can be predicted that those who argue that gerontology is not an academic discipline will be opposed to such programs.

A final and pressing issue of concern to academic gerontologists is the relationship between gerontology and geriatrics. The AGHE-USC national survey of gerontology instruction indicated a dramatic increase (17 percent) between 1976–1986 in the number of gerontology faculty who reported their departments of primary appointment to be in the health professions (Bolton, 1988). During this same period, faculty who reported their primary department appointment to be in gerontology declined by 10 percent (Bolton, 1988). The AGHE-USC survey also found that more than half (56 percent) of faculty respondents had no formal academic preparation in gerontology or geriatrics, with those in medical center settings having the least (32 percent) (Bolton, 1988). Publication rates, especially for journal articles related to gerontology/geriatrics, were strikingly higher among medical center faculty and had increased sharply since 1976 (Bolton, 1988). Along with these indications of recent growth in geriatrics, projections of the need for faculty and practitioners in health-related areas (NIA, 1984) dramatically illustrate the emergence of the health professions as a major new force in gerontology.

Historically, gerontologists and geriatricians have maintained their distances. Interactions between the two groups have often been characterized by poor communication, misunderstanding, and resentment. Neither has understood the other's disciplinary perspective or made much effort toward an understanding. Geriatrics has been primarily a developing field of practice, grounded in clinical and basic biomedical research. Gerontology has become an interdisciplinary science with emphasis on social, psychological, economic, and political as well as biological considerations. Gerontologists have recognized the role of health in the aging process and the need for interdisciplinary teamwork to satisfy elders' needs. Current concerns for meeting the chronic health care needs of an aging population have led health professionals to consider social and psychological issues and to implement interdisciplinary approaches to care. As Sauvageot (1978) noted, "To be a skilled geriatrician, one must be a good gerontologist and practice the skills of each discipline in treating patients" (p. 229).

The Long Term Care Gerontology Centers funded by the Administration on Aging, the Geriatric Education Centers established by the Bureau of Health Professions, and the Geriatric Research, Education and Clinical Centers of the Veterans Administration have provided organizational frameworks within which multidisciplinary collaborative relationships among geriatricians and gerontologists are required. Efforts begun through these units represent only beginning steps, and much remains to be done in order to overcome barriers and negotiate truly cooperative relationships. Much can be gained if health professionals and gerontologists learn to view each other as resources to be shared.

As dramatically presented in the 1987 report to Congress by the Department of Health and Human Services on personnel for health needs of the elderly through the year 2020 (NIA, 1987), the demand for aging service providers in all health disciplines will increase sharply. The demographics of an aging population have created an immediate need to grapple with the relationship between geriatrics and gerontology in educating health professionals.

As this practical reality is dealt with, gerontologists must also consider questions raised throughout the history of academic gerontology. The AGHE Standards Project represents a systematic effort to deal with some of these questions. In order for academic gerontology to move beyond the frontier and continue development as a professional field, the interdisciplinary issues require serious attention. Regardless of how these issues are resolved, educational gerontology's frontier will continue to be a promising and exciting one that will ultimately prove to be of benefit to students, educators, and older adults alike.

REFERENCES

Adler, M. (1958). History of Gerontological Society, Inc. *Journal of Gerontology, 13,* 94–102.

Administration on Aging (1976). Older Americans Act of 1965, as amended. Washington, D.C.: U.S. Department of Health, Education and Welfare.

Aging Research and Training News (1987, November 23).

American Psychological Association (1948). Report of the Committee on Instruction for Maturity and Old Age. Division of Maturity and Old Age.

American Psychological Association (1985). *A Guide to Doctoral Study in the Psychology of Adult Development and Aging.* Washington, D.C.: American Psychological Association.

Arling, G., and Romaniuk, J. G. (1980). *Final Report of the Task Force on Gerontology in Higher Education.* Richmond: Virginia Center on Aging.

Atchley, R. C. (1985). *Social Forces and Aging.* 4th ed. Belmont, Calif.: Wadsworth Publishing Co., Inc.

Birren, J. (Ed.) (1959). *Handbook of Aging and the Individual: Psychological and Biological Aspects.* Chicago: University of Chicago Press.

Bolton, C. R. (1988). The teachers of gerontology, 1976–1986. *AGHE Exchange,* 2 (2), 6–7.

Bolton, C. R., Eden, D. Z., Holcomb, J. R., and Sullivan, K. R. (1978). *Gerontology Education in the United States: A Research Report.* Omaha: University of Nebraska.

Bramwell, R. D. (1985). Gerontology as a discipline. *Educational Gerontology,* 11, 201–10.

Burgess, E. (Ed.) (1960). *Aging in Western Societies: A Survey of Social Gerontology.* Chicago: University of Chicago Press.

Byerts, T. O., and Taylor, P. S. (Eds.) (1977). Environment and aging. *Journal of Architectural Education,* 31.

Council on Social Work Education, Inc. (1964). *Teacher's Source Book on Aging.* New York: CSWE.

Craig, B. M. (1982). Weighing the issues and consequences of federal program termination: Administration on Aging support for career preparation. *Gerontology and Geriatrics Education,* 3, 129–37.

Danish, S. J. (1980). The land of help in the twentieth century. *Rutgers Professional Psychology Review,* 2, 24–25.

Danish, S. J., and Smyer, M. A. (1981). Unintended consequences of requiring a license to help. *American Psychologist,* 36, 13–21.

Donahue, W. (1960, November). Training in social gerontology. *Geriatrics,* 801–9.

Dressel, P. L., and Mayhew, L. B. (1974). *Higher Education as a Field of Study.* San Francisco: Jossey-Bass.

Education and training in gerontology—1970 (1970). *The Gerontologist,* 10, 53–72, 153–60.

Frank, L. K. (1946). Gerontology. *Journal of Gerontology,* 1, 1–11.

Ganikos, M. L. (Ed.) (1979). *Counseling the Aged: A Training Syllabus for Educators.* Washington, D.C.: United States Department of Health, Education and Welfare.

Gross, S. J. (1978, November). The myth of professional licensing. *American Psychologist,* 1009–16.

Hartford, M. E. (1980). Study of the vocational interests of the first two masters degree classes of the Leonard Davis School—1975 and 1976. *The Gerontologist,* 20, 526–33.

Hirschfield, I. S., and Peterson, D. A. (1982). The professionalization of gerontology. *The Gerontologist*, 22, 215–20.

Hogan, D. B. (1979). *The Regulation of Psychotherapists. Vol. I: A Study in the Philosophy and Practice of Professional Regulation.* Cambridge, Mass.: Ballinger.

Johnson, H. R. (1980). Introduction. In C. Tibbitts, H. Friedsam, P. Kerschner, G. Maddox, and H. McClusky. *Academic Gerontology: Dilemmas of the 1980's,* pp. 3–6. Ann Arbor: University of Michigan.

Johnson, H. R., Britton, J. H., Lang, C. A., Seltzer, M. M., Stanford, E. P., Yancik, R., Maklan, C., and Middleswarth, A. (1980). Foundations for gerontological education. *The Gerontologist*, 20, 1–61.

Kahl, A. (1976). Jobs with service programs. *Occupational Outlook Quarterly*, 20, 13–29.

Kane, R. L., Solomon, D. H., Beck, J. C., Keeler, E., and Kane, R. A. (1980). *Geriatrics in the United States: Manpower Projections and Training Considerations.* Santa Monica, Calif.: Rand Corporation.

Ketron, Inc. (1981). *Evaluation of the Title IV-A Career Training Program in Aging.* Washington, D.C.: Ketron, Inc.

Kleemeir, R. W. (1965). Gerontology as a discipline. *The Gerontologist*, 5, 237–39.

Kleemeir, R. W., Havighurst, R. J., and Tibbitts, C. (1967). Social gerontology. In R. E. Kushner and M. E. Bunch (Eds.), *Graduate Education in Aging within the Social Sciences,* pp. 37–52. Ann Arbor: University of Michigan, Division of Gerontology.

Koocher, G. P. (1979). Credentialing in psychology: Close encounters with competence? *American Psychologist*, 34, 696–702.

Krause, D. (1987). Careers in gerontology: Occupational fact or academic fantasy? *The Gerontologist*, 27, 30–33.

Kushner, R. E., and Bunch, M. W. (Eds.) (1967). *Graduate Education in Aging within the Social Sciences.* Ann Arbor: University of Michigan, Division of Gerontology.

Levine, M. (1981). Does gerontology exist? *The Gerontologist*, 21, 2–3.

Lobenstine, J. (Ed.) (1985). *National Directory of Educational Programs in Gerontology.* Washington, D.C.: Association for Gerontology in Higher Education.

Mangum, W. P., and Rich, T. A. (1980). Ten years of career training in gerontology: The University of South Florida experience. *The Gerontologist*, 20, 519–25.

Matarazzo, J. D. (1977, October). Higher education, professional accreditation and licensure. *American Psychologist*, 856–59.

Myers, J. E. (1983). Gerontological counseling training: The state of the art. *The Personnel and Guidance Journal*, 61, 398–401.

National Association of Social Workers (1983). Geriatrics social work picked as growth area. *NASW News*, 3.

National Clearinghouse on Aging (1976). *AOA Occasional Papers in Gerontology: No. 1 Manpower Needs in the Field of Aging: The Nursing Home Industry.* Washington, D.C.: U.S. Government Printing Office.

National Institute on Aging (1984). *Report on Education and Training in Geriatrics and Gerontology.* Washington, D.C.: National Institute on Aging, Public Health Service, U.S. Department of Health and Human Services.

National Institute on Aging (1987). *Personnel for Health Needs of the Elderly through Year 2020.* Washington, D.C.: Public Health Service, U.S. Department of Health and Human Services.

Nelson, G. M., and Schneider, R. L. (1984). *The Current Status of Gerontology in Graduate Work Education*. New York: Council on Social Work Education.

Niederehe, G. (1982). Postgraduate training of psychologists for work in aging: Continuing education, retraining, and services education. In J. F. Santos and G. R. VandenBos (Eds.), *Psychology and the Older Adult: Challenges for Training in the 1980's*. Washington, D.C.: American Psychological Association, Inc.

Peterson, D. A. (1978). An overview of gerontology education. In M. M. Seltzer, H. Sterns, and T. Hickey (Eds.), *Gerontology in Higher Education: Perspectives and Issues*, pp. 14–26. Belmont, Calif.: Wadsworth.

Peterson, D. A. (1984). Are master's degrees in gerontology comparable? *The Gerontologist*, 24, 646–51.

Peterson, D. A. (1985). Employment experience of gerontology master's degree graduates. *The Gerontologist*, 25, 514–19.

Peterson, D. A. (1987). *Career Paths in the Field of Aging: Professional Gerontology*. Lexington, Mass.: D. C. Heath.

Peterson, D. A., and Bolton, C. R. (1980). *Gerontology Instruction in Higher Education*. New York: Springer.

Peterson, D. A., Douglass, E. B., Bolton, C. R., Connelly, J. R., and Bergstone, D. (1987). *Gerontology Instruction in American Institutions of Higher Education: A National Survey*. Washington, D.C.: Association for Gerontology in Higher Education and the Andrus Gerontology Center, University of Southern California.

Rich, T. A., Giordano, J., Mullins, L. C., and Dunn, V. (1986). Curriculum of a third kind: Moving into a new age by degrees. Discussion session at the annual meeting of the Association for Gerontology in Higher Education, Atlanta, Georgia, February 27-March 2.

Ridley, J., Charlotte, L., Connelly, R., Albright, D., Pena, R., Gilford, R., Shirley, M. (1978, Summer). Draft standards and guidelines. *Generations*, 3, 44–51.

Santos, J. F., and VandenBos, G. R. (Eds.) (1982). *Psychology and the Older Adult: Challenges for Training in the 1980's*. Washington, D.C.: American Psychological Association.

Sauvageot, J. P. (1978). Gerontology and geriatrics in professional curricula of medical schools. In M. M. Seltzer, H. Sterns, and T. Hickey (Eds.), *Gerontology in Higher Education: Perspectives and Issues*, pp. 228–31. Belmont, Calif.: Wadsworth.

Seltzer, M. M. (1982). Academic gerontology program maintenance. *Gerontology and Geriatrics Education*, 3, 77–79.

Seltzer, M. M. (1983). A proposed sociology of gerontology. *Gerontology and Geriatrics Education*, 4, 3–9.

Seltzer, M. M. (1985). Issues of accreditation of academic gerontology programs and credentialing of workers in the field of aging. *Gerontology and Geriatrics Education*, 5, 7–18.

Seltzer, M. M., Sterns, H., and Hickey, T. (Eds.) (1978). *Gerontology in Higher Education: Perspectives and Issues*. Belmont, Calif.: Wadsworth Publishing Co., Inc.

Simson, S., and Wilson, L. B. (1981). The performance of Administration on Aging Multidisciplinary Gerontology Centers for Education and Training. *Educational Gerontology*, 7, 215–29.

Spence, D. L. (1983). Departments of gerontology? Toward significant survival. *Gerontology and Geriatrics Education,* 4, 5–14.

Sprouse, B. M. (Ed.) (1976). *National Directory of Educational Programs in Gerontology.* 1st ed. Washington, D.C.: Department of Health, Education and Welfare, Office of Human Development, Administration on Aging.

Sterns, H. L., Ansello, E. F., Sprouse, B. M., and Layfield-Faux, R. (Eds.) (1979). *Gerontology in Higher Education: Developing Institutional and Community Strength.* Belmont, Calif.: Wadsworth.

Storandt, M. (1978). Major concerns and future directions in gerontology and higher education: A perspective from our knowledge base. In M. M. Seltzer, H. Sterns, and T. Hickey (Eds.), *Gerontology in Higher Education: Perspectives and Issues,* pp. 38–45. Belmont, Calif.: Wadsworth Publishing Co., Inc.

Sullivan, E. (Ed.) (1982). *National Directory of Educational Programs in Gerontology.* Washington, D.C.: Association for Gerontology in Higher Education.

Tibbitts, C. (Ed.) (1960). *Handbook of Social Gerontology: Societal Aspects of Aging.* Chicago: University of Chicago Press.

Tibbitts, C. (1980). Training. In C. Tibbitts, H. Friedsam, P. Kershner, G. Maddox, and H. McClusky, *Academic Gerontology: Dilemmas of the 1980's,* pp. 9–24. Ann Arbor: University of Michigan.

U.S. Department of Health, Education and Welfare, Office on Aging (1965). *Training in Social Gerontology and its Applications.* Washington, D.C.: U.S. Government Printing Office.

University of Michigan Institute for Social Gerontology (1959). *Syllabi in Social Gerontology.* Ann Arbor: University of Michigan Institute for Social Gerontology.

Van Orman, R. (1984, March). Bachelor's degree curricula in gerontology. Paper presented at Western Gerontological Society Meeting, Anaheim, California.

Williams, E. (1987). *Opportunities in Gerontology Careers.* Lincolnwood, Ill.: VGM Career Horizons.

AUTHOR INDEX

SUBJECT INDEX

ABOUT THE CONTRIBUTORS

EVAN CALKINS was founding President of the Network in Aging of Western New York, Inc., and serves as the Director of the Western New York Geriatric Education Center. A member of numerous medical societies, he was recently elected Chair-elect of the clinical medical section of the Gerontological Society of America. He has served as President of the American Rheumatism Association, as a member of the Advisory Council on Aging, of the National Institute of Aging, and is recipient of the Milo D. Leabitt Award of the American Geriatric Society. He is editor or coeditor of four books, including *The Practice of Geriatrics* (1986) and *Principles and Practice of Nursing Home Care* (1988) and author of numerous scientific publications.

ANTHONY P. GLASCOCK is Professor of Anthropology and Head of the Psychology/Sociology/Anthropology Department at Drexel University. His research has focused on the treatment of the elderly in nonindustrial societies, and he has published numerous articles on the subject. He is currently analyzing data collected during fourteen months of research on old age and the aging process in two Irish communities. He has also conducted research on aging among agropastoralists in South Central Somalia. He received his Ph.D. from the University of Pittsburgh.

KAREN HOOKER is an Assistant Professor of Psychology at Syracuse University. Her research areas are personality and health in adulthood. She received her Ph.D. in Human Development and Family Studies from the Pennsylvania State University and subsequently was a Postdoctoral Fellow at the Duke University Center for the Study of Aging and Human Development.

BARBARA HORNUM is Assistant Professor of Anthropology at Drexel University. Her research has focused on the elderly in planned communities in the United States and Great Britain. Among her publications are articles on "Dependency Fears and Selection of Living Arrangements: A Study of One Life Care Community in America," "The Elderly and Alternative Options for Long-Term Care," "The Elderly in British New Towns," and "Aspects of Aging in Planned Communities." She received her Ph.D. from Bryn Mawr College.

WILLIAM J. HOYER is Professor of Psychology at Syracuse University and Associate, All-University Gerontology Center at Syracuse University. He is also adjunct Research Professor at SUNY Health Sciences Center at Syracuse. Hoyer is a Fellow of the Gerontological Society of America and a Fellow of the American Psychological Association. Hoyer's research area is the psychology of aging. His area of specialization is perceptual and cognitive functioning in middle and later adulthood. Hoyer received his Ph.D. in experimental and developmental psychology from West Virginia University.

ROSELLE KALOSIEH is a doctoral candidate in counseling psychology at Seton Hall University. She coordinated the guidance and counseling component of a systemwide project in career education sponsored by the federal government. Her research interests include cognitive styles, learning as a life-long process, and adult development and aging.

JURGIS KARUZA is an Assistant Director—Evaluation and Research of the Western New York Geriatric Education Center, Research Assistant Professor of Medicine, Division of Geriatrics/Gerontology, State University of New York at Buffalo, and Associate Professor of Psychology at the State University College at Buffalo. His research interests include evaluations of interdisciplinary networks and educational programs in geriatrics, investigation of the models of helping and coping used by elderly adults, examination of ethical and quality of care issues in geriatric primary and long-term care settings, and investigation of oral status and its impact on the well-being of older adults. He received his Ph.D. in Social Psychology from Wayne State University and a Specialist Certificate in the Psychology of Aging from University of Michigan–Wayne State University Institute of Gerontology.

LOUIS LOWY is Professor Emeritus at Boston University. He has pioneered gerontological social work since 1957 when he joined the university. He was cofounder of the Boston University Center of Gerontology in 1974. He engaged in many social welfare research projects and was actively involved in social work practice with the aging. He has authored six major books (including titles in German) and published over one hundred articles, largely in social gerontology, here and abroad. He received his Ph.D. from Harvard. A chair in social gerontology and social policy was established in his name at Boston University upon his retirement.

EDWARD J. MASORO has held faculty positions at Queen's University (Canada), Tufts University School of Medicine, University of Washington, and Medical College of Pennsylvania. Since 1973 he has been Professor and Chairman of the Department of Physiology at the University of Texas Health Science Center at San Antonio. His research has been in lipid metabolism, cold exposure, membrane biochemistry, and gerontology. Since 1975 his research has focused on influence of food restriction on aging. He has or is serving in an editorial role for: *J. Lipid Research; Experimental Aging Research; Experimental Gerontology; J. Gerontol.: Biol. Sciences; Growth, Development and Aging; Proc. Soc. Exper. Biol. Med.* He has served as Chairman of the Aging Review Committee of the NIA and is serving as Chairman of the Board of Scientific Counselors of the NIA. He received his Ph.D degree from the University of California at Berkeley.

NANCY J. OSGOOD is Associate Professor of Gerontology and Sociology at Virginia Commonwealth University/Medical College of Virginia in Richmond. For the past nine years she has been conducting research, writing, and teaching courses in the area of social gerontology. She is a former member of the National Committee on Vital and Health Statistics (NCVHS). Her main areas of research interest and expertise include suicide in the elderly, housing for the elderly, recreation, leisure, and aging, and substance abuse among the elderly. Osgood has authored several books including *Life After Work* (1982), *Senior Settlers* (1982), and *Suicide in the Elderly* (1985). She has published many articles in the field of gerontology. She received her Ph.D. in Sociology and her Certificate in Gerontology from Syracuse University.

IRIS A. PARHAM is Chairperson and Associate Professor of Gerontology, Virginia Commonwealth University, holds joint appointments in Geriatric Medicine and Psychology, and is Executive Director of the Geriatric Education Center at Virginia Commonwealth University, Richmond, Virginia. She has copublished two volumes of gerontology/geriatrics curriculum modules, which have been disseminated nationally. She is currently editor for a similar curriculum project being developed through the American Psychological Association and has published numerous articles on various psychological aspects of aging. Parham is also coauthor of *Crisis Intervention with the Elderly* (1988). She holds a Ph.D. in Developmental-Aging Psychology from the University of Southern California.

JOSEPH P. PEDOTO is a Counseling Psychology Ph.D. candidate at Seton Hall University. Formerly a clinical director at the Patrick House Drug Program and the Director of Counseling at Bergen Supported Work Program (a Ford Foundation project), he is now Director of the Educational Opportunity Fund Program at Hudson County Community College in Jersey City. Pedoto has previously written about the problems of the older adult as community college student and on the role of ethnicity in counseling.

ANN H.L. SONTZ is President of the Brunswick Institute, a research center devoted to inquiries on aging and human development studies. She has published on the status of immigrant family life within the European Economic Community and with the Pace University economist, Philip K.Y. Young, on midlife and older adult immigrants in small business enterprise in the United States. Sontz is the author of *Philanthropy and Gerontology: The Role of American Foundations* (Greenwood Press, 1989) and is currently at work on an historical study of academic philanthropy. Sontz holds a Ph.D. in Anthropology from Columbia University where she was nominated to a John W. Burgess Distinguished Fellowship.

JODI L. TEITELMAN is Assistant Professor in the Department of Gerontology and Training Director of the Geriatric Education Center at Virginia Commonwealth University, Richmond, Virginia. Teitelman has published in the areas of geriatrics education and training, late-life sexuality, and learned helplessness in the elderly. She is coeditor of the two-volume *Modular Gerontology Curriculum for Health Professionals* and coauthor of *Crisis Intervention with the Elderly* (1988), and the forthcoming *Late-Life Sexuality: Psychosocial Aspects of Function and Dysfunction*. She received both her doctorate in Psychology and a Certificate in Aging Studies from Virginia Commonwealth University.

JOAN B. WOOD is Assistant Professor in the Department of Gerontology and Education Services and Director of the Geriatric Education Center at Virginia Commonwealth University, Richmond, Virginia. Her research interests are focused on the dynamics of family caregiving, especially of Alzheimer's patients, and delivery of health care to older ethnic minorities. She has published in the areas of geriatrics education and training, age-related cognitive changes, and ethnic and minority issues in aging. She is the author of *Paraprofessional Home Care Providers in Multicultural Settings* and *Curriculum Modules in Minority Aging*. Wood received her Ph.D. in Developmental Psychology from Virginia Commonwealth University.